RECENT ADVANCES IN HEMATOLOGY RESEARCH

THROMBOTIC THROMBOCYTOPENIC PURPURA

CAUSES, DIAGNOSIS AND TREATMENT

RECENT ADVANCES IN HEMATOLOGY RESEARCH

Additional books and e-books in this series can be found on Nova's website under the Series tab.

RECENT ADVANCES IN HEMATOLOGY RESEARCH

THROMBOTIC THROMBOCYTOPENIC PURPURA

CAUSES, DIAGNOSIS AND TREATMENT

MASON HILLAM
EDITOR

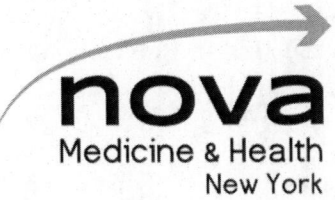

Copyright © 2019 by Nova Science Publishers, Inc.

All rights reserved. No part of this book may be reproduced, stored in a retrieval system or transmitted in any form or by any means: electronic, electrostatic, magnetic, tape, mechanical photocopying, recording or otherwise without the written permission of the Publisher.

We have partnered with Copyright Clearance Center to make it easy for you to obtain permissions to reuse content from this publication. Simply navigate to this publication's page on Nova's website and locate the "Get Permission" button below the title description. This button is linked directly to the title's permission page on copyright.com. Alternatively, you can visit copyright.com and search by title, ISBN, or ISSN.

For further questions about using the service on copyright.com, please contact:
Copyright Clearance Center
Phone: +1-(978) 750-8400   Fax: +1-(978) 750-4470   E-mail: info@copyright.com.

NOTICE TO THE READER

The Publisher has taken reasonable care in the preparation of this book, but makes no expressed or implied warranty of any kind and assumes no responsibility for any errors or omissions. No liability is assumed for incidental or consequential damages in connection with or arising out of information contained in this book. The Publisher shall not be liable for any special, consequential, or exemplary damages resulting, in whole or in part, from the readers' use of, or reliance upon, this material. Any parts of this book based on government reports are so indicated and copyright is claimed for those parts to the extent applicable to compilations of such works.

Independent verification should be sought for any data, advice or recommendations contained in this book. In addition, no responsibility is assumed by the Publisher for any injury and/or damage to persons or property arising from any methods, products, instructions, ideas or otherwise contained in this publication.

This publication is designed to provide accurate and authoritative information with regard to the subject matter covered herein. It is sold with the clear understanding that the Publisher is not engaged in rendering legal or any other professional services. If legal or any other expert assistance is required, the services of a competent person should be sought. FROM A DECLARATION OF PARTICIPANTS JOINTLY ADOPTED BY A COMMITTEE OF THE AMERICAN BAR ASSOCIATION AND A COMMITTEE OF PUBLISHERS.

Additional color graphics may be available in the e-book version of this book.

Library of Congress Cataloging-in-Publication Data

ISBN: 978-1-53615-353-8
Library of Congress Control Number: 2019937825

Published by Nova Science Publishers, Inc. † New York

CONTENTS

Preface		vii
Chapter 1	Causes and Risk Factors for Thrombotic Thrombocytopenic Purpura *Llanos Belmonte Andújar, Yanira Romero Sierra, Esther López del Cerro, Ana Dolores del Rey Luján and Carmen Cristina Amorós Pérez*	1
Chapter 2	Diagnosis of Thrombotic Thrombocytopenic Purpura *Ana Dolores Del Rey Luján, Carmen Cristina Amorós Pérez, Llanos Belmonte Andújar, Lorena Pico Rico and Martin Antonio Cabero Becerra*	29
Chapter 3	Differential Diagnosis and Treatment of Thrombotic Thrombocytopenic Purpura *Martin Antonio Cabero - Becerra, Lorena Picó Rico, Ana Dolores Del Rey Lujan, Carmen Cristina Amorós Pérez and Llanos Belmonte Andújar*	55

Chapter 4	Treatment of Thrombotic Thrombocytopenic Purpura during Pregnancy *A. Fuentes Rozalén, Y. Ben-Aïcha González and Ll. Belmonte Andújar*	**87**
Index		**101**
Related Nova Publications		**107**

PREFACE

Thrombotic thrombocytopenic purpura is a life-threatening occlusive disorder of the microcirculation that is characterized by systemic platelet agglutination, organ ischaemia, severe thrombocytopenia and fragmentation of red blood cells. In the opening study included in Thrombotic Thrombocytopenic Purpura: Causes, Diagnosis and Treatment, the authors analyze the principal risk factors and causes of this disorder.

Thrombotic thrombocytopenic purpura is diagnosed using standard laboratory tests: in addition to microangi-opathic hemolytic anemia and consumption thrombocytopenia, classical parameters for hemolysis show an elevated reticulocyte count, an undetectable serum haptoglobin concentration, and a markedly elevated lactate dehydrogenase level as well as the presence of schistocytes on the blood smear.

The authors propose that there are other pathologies with moderate thrombocytopenia that the authors should consider, such as: hereditary thrombotic thrombocytopenic purpura, hereditary hemolytic uremic syndrome, and thrombotic microangiopathies associated with some medications, transplantation or hidden malignancies.

The closing chapter aims to revise the management of thrombotic thrombocytopenic purpura in pregnant women. To effectively manage this disorder, it is crucial to obtain a prompt diagnosis, in conjunction with further monitoring and treatment, to avoid fetal loss and maternal complications.

Chapter 1 - Thrombotic thrombocytopenic purpura (TTP) is a life-threatening occlusive disorder of the microcirculation that is characterized by systemic platelet agglutination, organ ischaemia (especially of the brain, heart, gastrointestinal tract and kidneys), severe thrombocytopenia (a low blood platelet count, $<100 \times 10^9$ cells per litre, often $<30 \times 10^9$ cells per litre) and fragmentation of red blood cells. Although rare, TTP has the capacity to progress quickly, with 10% of mortality despite optimal management. During the last few years, different hypotheses have been considered, including genetic alterations that could cause a predisposition to TTP. The most common of theses alterations is an inherited or acquired deficiency of a metalloproteinase, which is an important and the only identified causing factor but nonessential for the development of TTP. Significant advances have taken place during the last decades in understanding the physiopathology of this disease, but there is still a certain degree of controversy in stablishing the limits that separate TTP from other clinical entities, mainly distinguishing its triggers from possible clearly separated entities. The objective of this chapter is to perform a review of the literature in order to analyze the principal risk factors and causes of Thrombotic thrombocytopenia purpura are and, if possible, their strength of association. The knowledge of these factors and causes would be interesting and useful for providing new prevention strategies, pharmacological and non-pharmacological, in order to reduce relapses and mortality of this rare disorder.

Chapter 2 - Thrombotic thrombocytopenic purpura (TTP) is a rare and life-threatening thrombotic microangiopathy characterized by micro-angiopathic hemolytic anemia, severe thrombocytopenia, and organ ischemia related to disseminated thrombosis. In 1924, TTP was first clinically described by Eli Moschcowitz in a 16-year-old girl as fatal thrombotic microangiopathy. Until the 1980s to 1990s, the etiology for TTP remained unknown. During the last few years, different hypotheses have been considered, including genetic alterations that could cause a predisposition to PTT, the most common: ADAMTS 13 mutations. TTP is twice as frequent in women, and its outcome is characterized by being prone to relapse. Rapid recognition of TTP is crucial to initiate appropriate treatment, without treatment, it leads to death in 90% of patients, often during the first 24 hours, mainly due to ischemic episodes. The incidence of acquired PTT is much higher in adults (2.9 cases /million/year) than in children (0.1 cases/ million/year). Acquired thrombotic thrombocytopenic purpura usually presents with an acute clinical course, with a tendency to relapse and occasional association of other autoimmune disorders. The classic clinical description of PTT has been the pentad of microangiopathic hemolytic anemia, thrombocytopenia, fever, renal failure and neurologic findings, but not all patients present it. The diagnosis of PTT is made by standard laboratory tests: In addition to the microangiopathic hemolytic anemia and consumption thrombocytopenia, classical parameters for hemolysis show an elevated reticulocyte count, an undetectable serum haptoglobin concentration, and a markedly elevated lactate dehydrogenase level as well as the presence of schistocytes on the blood smear. Direct antiglobulin (Coombs) test (DAT) is negative. Standard coagulation parameters are usually normal, but severe organ ischemia may cause disseminated intravascular coagulation, which is associated with coagulation abnormalities. Kidney assessment may show proteinuria, hematuria, and sometimes elevated plasma urea and creatinine levels. As these standard investigations are not specific for TTP, they must be accompanied by the assessment of ADAMTS13, the unique sensitive and specific marker for TTP. The specialized laboratories can determine 3 aspects related to ADAMTS13: antigen, activity and presence of antibodies. The ADAMTS13 activity is the main parameter to be evaluated due to its informative value regarding the functionality of the molecule.

Chapter 3 - Thrombotic thrombocytopenic purpura (TTP) is usually diagnosed with thrombocytopenia, microangiopathic hemolytic anemia, neuropathy, renal failure, and fever, although thrombocytopenia, schistocytes in the peripheral blood smear, and high levels of Lactic dehydrogenase (LDH) are sufficient for diagnosis. ADAMTS13 serum levels are very low and the coagulation study is usually normal, in contrast to other diseases. Thrombocytopenia of TTP is usually moderate, secondary to thrombotic microangiopathies (TMA). In addition, other pathologies may have moderate thrombocytopenia and must be differentiated. Indeed, the most frequent are hemolytic uremic syndrome associated with infection (HUS), HELLP syndrome and disseminated intravascular coagulation (DIC). There are other pathologies with moderate thrombocytopenia that the authors should consider, such as hereditary TTP, hereditary SHU, TMA associated with some medications, transplantation or hidden malignancies. The accuracy of the diagnosis is fundamental to be able to give the most effective treatment possible, to improve the long-term results. The usual treatment of autoimmune TTP is plasma exchange, using fresh frozen or cryoprecipitated plasma, eliminating vWF multimers of high molecular weight and providing ADAMTS13. In some cases, rituximab is effective in this condition, and the authors can use it together with the plasma exchange, which reduces the risk of relapse. In refractory cases, or in which relapse is frequent, high doses of corticosteroids, vincristine, intravenous immunoglobulin or immunosuppressive therapy, such as azathioprine or cyclophosphamide, would be used. In cases of HUS, renal support dialysis and control of hypertension are the pillars of the treatment. Platelet transfusions are contraindicated in HUS and TTP. For the atypical SUH, the treatment is similar to renal insufficiency, but the authors can add Eculizumab to inhibit the activation of the complement. Mortality is approximately 90% in non-treated cases for that reason a Clinical suspicion and a correct diagnosis is essential. The objective of this chapter is to indicate the most reliable tests collected from the literature, with the purpose of an early and accurate diagnosis, which is fundamental to administer the most appropriate treatment.

Chapter 4 - Thrombotic thrombocytopenic purpura (TTP), also known as Moschcowitz disease, is a rare but potentially life-threatening disorder that may affect childbearing age women. TTP is identified by concomitant occurrence of severe thrombocytopenia, microangiopathic haemolytic anemia and ischemic organ damage, particularly affecting the brain, heart and kidneys. The clinical features associated with TTP include microangiopathic hemolytic anemia, thrombocytopenia, neurological and renal alterations and fever. Genetic modifications could be associated with predisposition to suffer from TTP. Seventy-six mutations of ADAMTS 13 gene have been reported in the literature. As a consequence a deficiency of a disintegrin and metalloprotease with thrombospondin1-like domains (ADAMS13) is found. This deficiencyis involved in the production of normal von Willebrand factor multimers by cleaving the large multimers produced in endomthelial cells. ADAMS13 inefficiency leads to an accumulation of ULVWf, which induces platelet aggregation in the microvasculature, leading to thrombosis. Hence, resulting inmicro-angiopathic thrombosis and hemolysis. TTP is a medical emergency that can affect a wide range of ages (from 20 to 50 years old) and can be fatal if is not well diagnosed and appropriate treated thereafter. From 2.17 to 6 TTP cases per million are identified each year, from those TTP patients 12% up to 31% are associated with pregnancy. It must be remarked that women with TTP represent two-thirds of the affected patients. As mentioned, TTP not specific to pregnancy, but occurs with an increased frequency during pregnancy. A delay in the diagnosis of TTP during pregnancy may result in life-threatening maternal and fetal consequences, for that an urgent plasma-based therapy is needed. Therapeutic plasma Exchange (TPE) is the gold standard therapy, it consists on replenishing the depleted levels of ADAMTS13 and removing anti-ADAMTS13 antibodies. However, corticosteroids are also widely used to treat TTP, even though the benefits have not been shown conclusively. Delivery does not generally cause TTP resolution. For all, the purpose of this chapter is to revise de management of TTP in pregnant women. It is crucial to ensure a correct management by prompt diagnosis, monitoring and treatment to avoid its impact on fetal loss and maternal complications.

In: Thrombotic Thrombocytopenic Purpura ISBN: 978-1-53615-353-8
Editor: Mason Hillam © 2019 Nova Science Publishers, Inc.

Chapter 1

CAUSES AND RISK FACTORS FOR THROMBOTIC THROMBOCYTOPENIC PURPURA

Llanos Belmonte Andújar[1,*], *MD*,
Yanira Romero Sierra[1], *MD*,
Esther López del Cerro[2], *MD*,
Ana Dolores del Rey Luján[3], *MD*
and *Carmen Cristina Amorós Pérez*[4], *MD*

[1]Obstetrics and Gynecology Department,
Hospital of Almansa, Albacete, Spain
[2]Obstetrics and Gynecology Department,
Hospital of Gandía, Valencia, Spain
[3]Hematology and Hemotherapy, Hospital of Alcázar de San Juan,
Ciudad Real, Spain
[4]Hematology and Hemotherapy, Hospital Virgen de los Lirios,
Alcoy, Alicante, Spain

---

* Corresponding Author's E-mail: belmonte.llanos@gmail.com.

ABSTRACT

Thrombotic thrombocytopenic purpura (TTP) is a life-threatening occlusive disorder of the microcirculation that is characterized by systemic platelet agglutination, organ ischaemia (especially of the brain, heart, gastrointestinal tract and kidneys), severe thrombocytopenia (a low blood platelet count, $<100 \times 10^9$ cells per litre, often $<30 \times 10^9$ cells per litre) and fragmentation of red blood cells (Kremer Hovinga et al. 2017). Although rare, TTP has the capacity to progress quickly, with 10% of mortality despite optimal management (Marie Scully et al. 2012).

During the last few years, different hypotheses have been considered, including genetic alterations that could cause a predisposition to TTP. The most common of theses alterations is an inherited or acquired deficiency of a metalloproteinase, which is an important and the only identified causing factor but nonessential for the development of TTP (Page et al. 2016).

Significant advances have taken place during the last decades in understanding the physiopathology of this disease, but there is still a certain degree of controversy in stablishing the limits that separate TTP from other clinical entities, mainly distinguishing its triggers from possible clearly separated entities (Chang 2018).

The objective of this chapter is to perform a review of the literature in order to analyze the principal risk factors and causes of Thrombotic thrombocytopenia purpura are and, if possible, their strength of association. The knowledge of these factors and causes would be interesting and useful for providing new prevention strategies, pharmacological and non-pharmacological, in order to reduce relapses and mortality of this rare disorder.

Keywords: thrombotic thrombocytopenic purpura, TTP, Upshaw-Schulman syndrome, USS, risk factor, causes, ADAMTS13

INTRODUCTION

TTP was firstly clinically described by Eli Moschcowitz in 1924 in a 16-year-old female as a fatal thrombotic microangiopathy (TMA) including weakness, fever, transient focal neurologic symptoms, severe thrombocytopenia, and a microangiopathic hemolytic anemia linked to the presence of the terminal arterioles and capillaries (Moschcowitz 1925). In

1964, Amorosi and Ultmann published a review of all cases known to date and introduced the "classic pentad" used to diagnose TTP (Amorosi E.L., Ultmann J. E. 1966):

- Microangiopathic hemolytic anemia,
- Thrombocytopenia (with purpura),
- Acute kidney injury,
- Neurologic abnormality and fluctuating mental status, and
- Fever.

Nevertheless, its origin persisted undisclosed until Moake *et al.* in the early 1980s reported four cases of patients with chronic relapsing TTP who lacked the capacity to process von Willebrand factor (vWF) confirmed by the presence of plasma ultralarge vVW multimers hyperadhesive to platelets (Moake et al. 1982). During the mid-late 1990s, other investigators demonstrated that this inability to cleave vWF was the result of a severe deficiency of a metalloprotease (Furlan 2000)(Tsai and Lian 1998) which was later identified as *A Disintegrin And Metalloproteinase with Thrombospondin Motifs 13 (ADAMTS13)* and identified as the protein with vWF-cleaving activity that was deficient or absent in TTP.

Ultra-large vWF multimers are normally released from endothelial cells, and then cleaved by ADAMTS13 into smaller fragments which are important in primary haemostasis. In TTP, severely reduced ADAMTS13 activity allows uncleaved, ultra-large vWF multimers to accumulate in the microcirculation, where they bind and activate platelets causing microtrobi that obstruct the circulation in vital organs, causing thrombotic microangiopathy (TMA) (Fox et al. 2018). Consequently, TTP is defined as a TMA with severely reduced of ADAMTS13 activity, defined as a level under 10% of the normal enzyme activity) (Kremer Hovinga et al. 2017).

TMA is a pathologic diagnosis made by tissue biopsy. However, it is commonly inferred from the observation of microangiopathic hemolytic anemia (MAHA) and thrombocytopenia in the appropriate clinical setting. Acquired TTP was the first primary TMAs to be described and is perhaps the best understood of the TMAs regarding its pathophysiologically (George JM, Cuker A. 2018c).

The estimated annual incidence of TTP ranges from 3 to 11 cases per million residents per year (Terrell et al. 2005).

To discriminate TTP from other TMAs can be extremely complex, but its early diagnosis and urgent treatment with plasmapheresis are crucial to reduce the morbidity and mortality rates. Therefore, is very important to identify risk factors or probable triggers and take them into account in order to achieve the correct diagnosis.

THROMBOTIC THROMBOCYTOPENIC PURPURA: CLASSIFICATION

There are two main types of TTP according to whether the reduced enzyme activity setting is acquired or congenital:

- Congenital TTP (Upshaw-Schulman syndrome). Is due to ADAMTS13 mutations and responsible for <5% of TTP cases, in absence of inhibitory autoantibodies. The onset of the disease occurs at any age, with episodes often triggered by pregnancy/postpartum or infection.
- Acquired TTP. It results from the production of anti-ADAMTS13 auto-antibodies, and affects predominantly young women, although it can appear at any age, also its relative incidence is increased in people of black ethnicity (Terrell et al. 2005)(Joly et al. 2016)(Reese et al. 2013). This group represents the majority of cases of TTP (approximately 95%). Depending on its origin, acquired TTP may be:
  - Idiopatic: when the cause of TTP is ignored and there is not known underlying or associated condition.
  - Secondary: when the development of TTP is due to a predisposing or precipitating factor.

VON WILLEBRAND FACTOR

VWF is a plasma glycoprotein of 2050 amino acid residues, synthesized by endothelial cells and megakaryocytes (Verweij et al. 1986), which mediates platelet adhesion at sites of vascular injury. Its multimers are composed of identical subunits that are linked together by disulfide bonds. Each subunit consists of several kinds of repeated structural domains, and has binding sites for components of connective tissue, such as collagen, platelet membrane glycoproteins, factor VIII, and ADAMTS13 (Sadler 2017).

As described before, vWF is released from endothelial cells as ultralarge multimers, and ADAMTS13 progressively reduces the size of these VWF multimers as they circulate in the blood. Without a correct ADAMTS13 activity, these multimers eventually cause microtrombi. These disseminated microthrombi collect platelets, which causes thrombocytopenia, mechanically destroy red blood cells, which leads to haemolytic anaemia with fragmented red blood cells (schistocytes that are visible on the peripheral blood smear) and finally being able to embolize and occlude downstream arterioles causing tissue ischemia and infarctation of vital organs (Kremer Hovinga et al. 2017).

ADAMTS13

ADAMTS proteins are a superfamily of 26 secreted molecules comprising two related, but distinct families. ADAMTS proteases are zinc metalloendopeptidases, where most of its substrates are extracellular matrix components (Mead and Apte 2018). ADAMTS13 is primarily synthesized by stellate cells of the liver, renal podocytes and tubullar epithelial cells, platelets and vascular endothelial cells (Manea et al. 2010)(Liu et al. 2005)(Turner et al. 2006) and megakaryocytes, then secreted into plasma, after folding in the endoplasmic reticulum (Zander, Cao, and Zheng 2015)(Shelat, Ai, and Zheng 2005), where proteolyzes ultra-large von

Willebrand factor (vWF) multimers (ULvWF) at the Tyr1605-Met1606 bond in the A2 domain (Zheng, Majerus, and Sadler 2002), avoiding production of microtrombi by vWF and platelet aggregation.

The plasma concentration of ADAMTS 13 in humans ranges from 0.5 to 1.42 µg/ml, varying from different regions in the world (Miyata et al. 2013), its half-life in plasma is of 2-3 days (Furlan et al. 1999), and there is no known physiological inhibitor of this metalloproteinase´s activity. Although its activity is diminished in most patients with acute TTP, modest reductions may occur in a variety of medical conditions such as sepsis or liver disease and are not thought to cause clinical disease (George JM, Cuker A. 2018c). However, a single severe deficiency of ADAMTS13 activity is not enough to provoke TTP. Approximately half of the patients with hereditary ADAMTS13 deficiency do not present symptoms of TTP until adulthood, so it is thought that additional factors such as an acute inflammatory or prothrombotic stimulus (pregnancy, cancer, drugs, solid organ transplant or autoimmune disease) could act as triggers of clinical manifestations of TTP (George JM, Cuker A. 2018c).

It is known, also, that different enzymes apart from ADAMTS13 (leukocyte proteases, plasmin, granzyme and trombine), can replace its function of cleaving ultralarge vWF multimers, preventing the development of thrombosis in patients with severe ADAMTS13 deficiency (Chauhan 2014) (Tersteeg et al. 2014) (Kremer Hovinga et al. 2017), which could give rise to developing of new possible treatment options in the future.

As previously stated, there are two main types of TTP, congenital and acquired, that are described as follows:

CONGENITAL TTP

Hereditary TTP, also known as Upshaw-Schulman syndrome (USS), congenital TTP or familial TTP, is an autosomal recessive disease, in which patients have a severe ADAMTS13 deficiency, mostly complete absence of it, due to an inherited ADAMTS13 mutations (less than 5% of normal levels) (George JM, Cuker A. 2018b). Both alleles of the ADAMTS13 gene must be disrupted to suffer the clinical syndrome. USS is more often caused by compound heterozygous than homozygous mutations (Schneppenheim et al. 2006).

Congenital TTP was firstly described by Shulman (Schulman et al. 1960) in 1960 and Upshaw (Upshaw 1978) in 1978, but it was not until 2001, when Levy et al. (Levy et al. 2001) conducted linkage analysis of four bloodlines with congenital TTP, demonstrating that mutations in ADAMTS13 resulted in severely reduced vWF-cleaving protease activity in plasma, because of its impaired secretion.

The ADAMTS13 gene is located on chromosome 9q34, contains 29 exons, and en- codes a multidomain protein of 1427 amino acids. Over 150 different ADAMTS13 mutations have been identified worldwide. The mutations are distributed throughout the whole ADAMTS13 gene and consist of missense mutations (~70%), truncating mutations and insertions (~20%), as well as nonsense and splice site mutations (Hanby and Zheng 2014)(Taleghani et al. 2013).

Most of the mutations are restricted to entire families and homozygous cases are found mainly in patients with consanguineous background, but there are different mutations that predominate in Europe, Japan and other countries.

There are two predominating mutations: the single base insertion 4143insA in exon 29 and the missense mutation Arg1060Trp in exon 24, both have been observed in few unrelated families over an extensive geographic area. Whereas the single base insertion 4143insA appear to congregate around the Baltic sea (in Scandinavia and Moravia), the Arg1060Trp mutation has been observed in the United States and in many European countries (Kremer Hovinga et al. 2017).

Prevalence of USS is still unknown, but there are some estimations that calculate rates than range from 1.5 cases/million people in Oklahoma (EEUU), to 16.7 cases/million people in Norway (Europe)(von Krogh et al. 2016). Nowadays, there is a registry of patients with USS, and based on the publications of cases it is estimated that there are 150 families affected in the world. However, some authors postulate that USS could be more prevalent than predicted due to the occurrence of homozygous mutations in unrelated families, growing cases of affected patients who developed clinical disease during adulthood or remain asynmptomatic until old age, and the vast geographical areas of certain ADAMTS13 mutations (Taleghani et al. 2013) (Furlan and Lämmle 2001).

As mentioned above, in 2006, was created an international Hereditary TTP Registry (www.ttpregistry.net; ClinicalTrial.gov identifier: NCT01257269), with more than 130 patients and family members from 12 nations enrolled so far. The purpose of this registry is to gather further information and insight into this rare disease, eventually helping to improve the clinical management of affected patients. Inclusion of each new patient or family in this registry is crucial for investigation of new treatments, prophylactic measures, and risk/trigging factors identification, in order to avoid or reduce incidence and development of acute TTP in people affected by ADAMTS mutations.

Risk Factors for Congenital TTP/Upshaw-Schulman Syndrome

- *Age.* Between 30% and 50% of patients affected by USS developed their first episode of clinical TTP as early as their first days of life or before the age of five years, being called as early onset USS (Furlan and Lämmle 2001). Meanwhile, the other half of patients, as we described above, remain asymptomatic for decades until they present their first acute episode, frequently triggered by different identified risk factors, such as pregnancy, alcohol intoxication, infections, physiologic stress, drugs, and other unidentified genetic factors.
- *Race.* There does not appear to be any ethnic or racial difference in prevalence of congenital TTP.
- *Sex.* There is no sex disparity among patients diagnosed in infancy or childhood (Y. Fujimura et al. 2011). But, in patients diagnosed in adulthood, women are more frequently affected than men, relating to the fact that pregnancy is a known precipitating factor for an acute episode of TTP (George JM, Cuker A. 2018b).

- *Pregnancy.* Pregnancy, undoubtedly, is a strong inducer of TTP in female USS-patients, although the pathogenesis is not completely clarify. Actually, among women who suffered an episode of TTP during their first pregnancy, 25-66% of them were congenital TTP (Moatti-Cohen et al. 2012) (M. Scully et al. 2014). Different case reports documents have been published describing series of patients from families with severe constitutional vWF-cleaving protease deficiency, where pregnancy was a very frequent condition that induced fatal acute TTP in women, while men of the same family with the same severe vWF-cleaving protease deficiency were still asymptomatic at the age of 40 (Furlan and Lämmle 2001) (Kentouche et al. 2013) (Yoshihiro Fujimura et al. 2009). A study published in 2008 showed a relation with the missense ADAMPTS13 mutation p. R1060W and this late-onset TTP in pregnant women (Camilleri et al. 2008). Other studies show a major proportion of patients affected by TTP being pregnant women, compared with the general adulthood-onset percentage (Y. Fujimura et al. 2011) (Moatti-Cohen et al. 2012). A review by George in 2003 (George 2003), concluded that "pregnancy as a precipitating event for acute episodes of TTP-HUS is clear from many case series, including reports of women with congenital TTP-HUS. Pregnancy may be a risk factor for acute episodes of TTP-HUS because of the association of pregnancy with increasing concentrations of procoagulant factors, decreasing fibrinolytic activity, loss of endothelial cell thrombomodulin, and decreasing activity of ADAMTS13. All of these abnormalities become progressively more severe through the course of pregnancy, with the maximum abnormalities occurring at delivery and immediately postpartum". Since pregnancy is considered as a risk factor in acute inherited TTP, there is an important risk of relapse in subsequent pregnancies without prophylaxis (M. Scully et al. 2014).
- *Heavy alcohol intake.* A study analyzing the natural history of 43 USS-patients in Japan, concluded that alcohol intoxication could be

a strong trigger inducing TTP in this patients (Y. Fujimura et al. 2011).
- *Infections.* Certain *in vitro* studies show that infection and inflammation increase cytokines levels that promote release of vWF from human endothelial cells, and also inhibition of protelolytic cleavage of vWF by ADAMTS13 (Bernardo et al. 2004)(Pillai et al. 2016). Both factors could contribute significantly to the development of congenital or acquired TTP.
  - Influenza. The same Japanese study mentioned above shows that influenza infection could act as a trigger for TTP in USS patients (Y. Fujimura et al. 2011).
- *Drugs.* Different drugs, like desmopressin and interferon (Y. Fujimura et al. 2011), appear to be risk factors for developing TTP in patients with congenital deficiency of ADAMTS13, although with low evidence level.

Possible Modifying Factors

- *AB0 blood group.* The AB0 blood group gene is located near the ADAMTS13 gene. According to certain studies, some ADAMTS13 mutations such as T339R and P618A are associated with the blood group A allele, and other like P475S and S903L are associated with blood group 0 allele (Miyata et al. 2013).

Certainly, it is very complicated to establish the strength of association of all this possible risk factors or triggers with congenital TTP, due to the lack of frequency of this disease and the many possible undiagnosed patients that may exist. Further research might be necessary to deepen our knowledge of this rare disease and its risk and precipitating factors, taking into consideration the greatest importance of the inclusion of all newly diagnosed cases in the corresponding registries in order to conduct new studies on this matter.

ACQUIRED TTP

Acquired or idiophatic TTP is characterized by the appearance of auto-antibodies against ADAMTS13 that can either inhibit this metalloproteinase or not. It constitutes the majority of cases of TTP (approximately 95%), and its incidence is approximately three cases/million adults/year, based on data from the Oklahoma TTP-HUS Registry (Reese et al. 2013).

According to the review published by Kremer Hovinga in 2017, in most patients, strong functional ADAMTS13 inhibitors (mainly IgG class, IgM and IgA, less frequently) can be demonstrated. However, 10–25% of patients have non-inhibitory anti-ADAMTS13 auto-antibodies, which have been postulated to accelerate ADAMTS13 clearance, which could be an important contributing mechanism to reduce protease activity (Kremer Hovinga et al. 2017).

There are different conditions which appear to reduce ADMATS13 activity, although they are extremely unlikely to lower its activity to a disease-causing level. Moreover, ADAMTS13 activity also may be reduced by increasing of vWF levels, due to its consumption. These further reductions in ADAMTS13 activity and/or inflammatory stimuli in a patient with an underlying anti-ADAMTS13 autoantibody or hereditary ADAMTS13 deficiency may act as triggers for an acute episode of secondary TTP (George JM, Cuker A. 2018c).

The demographic characteristics and variability on the course of ADAMTS13 deficiency suggests that different factors, in the patient or the environment, influence the risk of developing TTP (Sadler 2017). Multiple factors have been proposed but their supporting evidence is variable.

Risk Factors for Acquired TTP

- *Age.* TTP mainly affects adults, with maximum incidence in the third of fifth decades of life in Europe and the United States (Kremer Hovinga et al. 2017). The median age for acquired TTP diagnosis is

41, with a wide range (9 to 78 years) (George JM, Cuker A. 2018a), being very infrequent among people younger than 18 years of age.
- *Sex distribution.* TTP Affects predominantly young women, with female to male ratios ranging from 2.5:1 to 3.5:1, although it can present at any age (Terrell et al. 2005)(Joly et al. 2016)(Reese et al. 2013)(Marie Scully et al. 2008). This could be related to the higher prevalence of other autoimmune conditions in women.
- *Race.* The relative incidence of TTP is increased in people of black ethnicity (Terrell et al. 2005)(Joly et al. 2016)(Reese et al. 2013), as well as other autoimmune diseases.

Possible Triggers Associated to Acquired Secondary TTP

- Acquired:
  - *Inflammation/Infection.* As stated in section of "Risk factors for congenital TTP", inflammation and infection could act increasing vWF levels and impairing ADAMTS 13 proteolytic activity, fostering the development of TTP. Hence, systemic bacterial, viral or fungal infections can cause and trigger TTP. On the other hand, some systemic infections can mimic the clinical characteristics of PTT presentation. According to Booth *et al,* the documentation of the severe deficiency of ADAMTS13 activity or the presence of an ADAMTS13 inhibitor does not exclude the existence of a systemic infection that mimics PTT. Certainly, in some cases could be difficult to differentiate whether the infection acts as the cause or the trigger (Booth et al. 2011).

Several types of infection have been reported related to TTP:

- *Pancreatitis.* The acute inflammatory response to pancreatitis may trigger the onset of TTP. One possible mechanism involves diffuse endothelial injury mediated by inflammatory cytokines that are released as part of the systemic inflammatory response to acute pancreatitis (Bergmann et al. 2008). However, few cases are published in the literature suggesting this disease as a triggering of real acute TTP with ADAMTS13 below 10% of its normal activity.

- *Sepsis:*
  - Capnocytophaga canimorsus (Smeets et al. 2018)(Brichacek, Blake, and Kao 2012). There are multiple case reports describing TTP secondary to c. Canimorsus sepsis, but as in most of the cases antibiotherapy (without plasmapheresis) solved the problem, is difficult to elucidate if the infection mimicked or caused real TTP.
- *Virus.* Viruses apparently are etiologic agents in the pathogenesis of TMA. Some might induce TTP while others are only associated with HUS. The exact pathophysiology of viral-associated TMA remains to be elucidated. However, direct endohelial cell injury appears to play an important role (Lopes da Silva 2011). Among the viruses related to TTP are:
  - *Human immunodeficiency virus* (HIV). HIV is the most common virus precipitating TTP (Opie 2012). This happens depending on the geographical area, the prevalence of the infection and also the availability of antiretroviral therapy. But is generally seen in patients with advanced disease and deeply low CD4 lymphocite count (<100 cells/mL) (Brecher, Hay, and Park 2008).
  - Other virus (Parvovirus B19, Dengue (Bastos et al. 2018), Chikungunya (Bastos et al. 2018), Influenza (Kosugi et al. 2010)(A and P 2015), Viral hepatitis, HTLV-1, Crimean-Congo fever virus, HHV-6 and 8, etc.) have been described in the literature as triggers of TTP, but there is not enough evidence to discriminate them as possible causes versus TTP mimickers.
  - *Autoimmune diseases/connective tissue disorders.* TTP can happen in patients affected by autoimmune and connective tissue disorders, mainly systemic lupus erythematosus (SLE) (Hamasaki et al. 2003), rheumatoid arthritis, and less frequent,

systemic esclerosis, scleroderma, dermatomyositis (Suzuki et al. 2013), Sjögren syndrome (Xu et al. 2018)(Yamashita et al. 2013) and also possibly in Grave´s (Chitnis et al. 2017) and Still´s disease (Sayarlioglu et al. 2008). In such cases, they would be TTP secondary to these disorders. However, the concomitant occurrence of TTP and these diseases is really uncommon, hence no clinical studies are possible in order to elucidate their connection. According to a recent epidemiological study, 75% of ADAMTS-13 activity deficiency is induced by anti-ADAMTS-13 IgG, which is potentially caused by underlying autoimmune diseases (Hamasaki et al. 2003). Also, autoantibodies characteristic of SLE have been detected in patients with acute TTP who have severe ADAMTS13 deficiency (George, Vesely, and James 2007).

- *Pregnancy.* The first report relating pregnancy with TTP was published in 1955 by Minner (Miner, Nutt, and Thomas 1955). Subsequently, many are the related documents published in this regard, which support the expectation of pregnancy acting as a trigger of TTP. Different TTP registries point out a clear relation between pregnancy and development of TTP in their statistics, and show as associated conditions along with pregnancy, ovarian stimulation, viral infection, thyroiditis, HIV, lupus or anti-phospholipid syndrome (Moatti-Cohen et al. 2012). As described before, once ADAMTS13 decrease its activity, levels of vWF increases, mainly due to consumption or related to estrogen from the second trimester on (Marie Scully et al. 2012). TTP could happen at any time during pregnancy and also during postpartum period. Acquired TTP probably occurs more frequently in pregnant women. Having suffered TTP during a previous pregnancy does not appear to increase the risk of TTP recurrence significantly during the next pregnancy, being uncommon the relapses with pregnancy following recovery from TTP. However acquired TTP during pregnancy may increase the frequency of preeclampsia and severe preeclampsia in subsequent pregnancies (Jiang et al. 2014) and also increases the risk of preeclampsia

o *Disseminated neoplasia.* Several case reports have been published about cancer relating to TTP, mainly those describing metastatic cancer. However, cancer barely causes real TTP with ADAMTS13 below 10% of the normal enzyme activity due to the presence of autoantibodies against this protease (George 2011). Most of the times these patients present microangiopathic hemolytic anemia and thrombocytopenia due to systemic microvascular metastases and bone marrow involvement, and also moderate decreases of ADMATS13 activity, similar to moderate ADAMTS13 deficiency that take place in multiple other disorders associated with systemic inflammation (infection, surgery, transplant, etc...). These clinical presentations mostly are confused and misdiagnosed as idiopathic TTP (Morton and George 2016)(Saha, McDaniel, and Zheng 2017).

o *Solid organ/marrow bone transplant.* There is no evident association between transplant and TTP, but as with disseminated neoplasia, ADAMTS13 levels could be diminished in such inflammatory processes. However, there are some case reports describing severe ADAMTS13 deficiency after lung transplant (Mal et al. 2006).

o *Drugs.* Two systematic reviews published in 2015 conclude that, although there are many case reports describing potential drug-induced TTP, there have been no cases of proven decreased ADMATS13 activity as the identified mechanism of TTP (Al-Nouri et al. 2015)(Reese et al. 2015). An exception to this would be the case of *Ticlopidine,* an antiplatelet drug of the thienopyridine family, which has been linked to development of acute TTP after 2-4 weeks of intake, affecting 1:1600 to 1:5000 patients who receive it (Tsai et al. 2000)(Bennett et al. 2013).

- Inherited:
  - HLA-DRB1*11: in some studies, this allele of the major histocompatibility complex class II gene family is apparently more related to acquired TTP in white people. While the allele HLA-DRB1*04 is suggested to be a possible protective factor in this disease's development (Coppo et al. 2010)(John, Hitzler, and Scharrer 2012). In fact, the low prevalence of this last allele in black population could be related with the higher prevalence of TTP in people of this ethnicity (Martino et al. 2016).
  - Heterozygosus ADAMTS13 mutations: according to different published case reports, this mutations could trigger the development of anti-ADAMTS13 autoantibodies or expedite a decrease in ADAMTS13 activity below a critical threshold and developed an acute TTP episode (De Cock et al. 2015)(Meyer, S. C. et al. 2007)

Possible Modifying Factors

- Individual variability in levels of glycoprotein I. The group of researchers leaded by Du, published in 2012 a report in which they described the relation between β_2GPI and TTP. This glycoprotein blocks platelet adhesion to endothelial cell-derived vWF strings. They concluded that levels of β_2GPI in plasma decreases significantly during an acute TTP episode, suggesting that β_2GPI may protect from the effects of hyper-functional VWF by inhibiting its interaction with platelets (Du et al. 2012). This finding glimpse a possible novel therapeutic approach for TTP.

As well as in congenital TTP, is very complicated to establish the exact connection between acquired TTP and its possible triggers or risk factors, due to the low prevalence of this condition. Further research might be necessary to improve the knowledge of this disease and to develop new strategies of prevention, early diagnosis and proper and prompt treatment, in order to reduce its mortality.

CONCLUSION

TTP is a rare condition resulting from ADAMTS13 severe deficiency, that can be either congenital (because of ADAMTS 13 gene mutations that produce ADAMTS13 deficiency or complete absence) or acquired (due to the production of anti-ADAMTS13 auto-antibodies).

Congenital TTP appears in half of the patients during the first days of life or before the age of five years (early onset disease). In the other half of patients, it usually develops in adulthood triggered by different factors like pregnancy, heavy alcohol intake, drugs or infections.

Acquired TTP usually appears in adulthood, during the third or fifth decade of life, being more frequent in women and people of black ethnicity.

Acquired TTP can be idiopathic (not related to other conditions or diseases) or secondary (triggered by other, known or not known, pathological situations: pregnancy, neoplasia, infections, inflammation, solid organ transplant or autoimmune diseases).

The rareness of both conditions (congenital and acquired TTP) does not allow the development of clinical trials and powerful research that could characterize the relationship between TTP and its possible risk factors or triggers.

Further research and the inclusion of every newly diagnosed case in the TTP registries are critical for the comprehension and study of both diseases.

REFERENCES

Al-Nouri, Zayd L., Jessica A. Reese, Deirdra R. Terrell, Sara K. Vesely, and James N. George. 2015. "Drug-Induced Thrombotic Microangi-opathy:

A Systematic Review of Published Reports." *Blood* 125 (4): 616–18. https://doi.org/10.1182/blood-2014-11-611335.

Amorosi E. L., Ultmann J. E. 1966. "Thrombotic Thrombocytopenic Purpura: Report of 16 Cases and Review of the Literature." *Medicine* 46 (2): 139–59.

Bastos, Maria Luiza Almeida, Ruth Maria Oliveira de Araújo, Deivide de Sousa Oliveira, Ana Nery Melo Cavalcante, and Geraldo Bezerra da Silva Junior. 2018. "Thrombotic Thrombocytopenic Purpura Associated with Dengue and Chikungunya Virus Coinfection: Case Report during an Epidemic Period." *Revista Do Instituto De Medicina Tropical De Sao Paulo* 60: e48. https://doi.org/10.1590/s1678-9946201860048.

Bennett, Charles L., Sony Jacob, Brianne L. Dunn, Peter Georgantopoulos, X. Long Zheng, Hau C. Kwaan, June M. McKoy, et al. 2013. "Ticlopidine-Associated ADAMTS13 Activity Deficient Thrombotic Thrombocytopenic Purpura in 22 Persons in Japan: A Report from the Southern Network on Adverse Reactions (SONAR)." *British Journal of Haematology* 161 (6): 896–98. https://doi.org/10.1111/bjh.12303.

Bergmann, I. P., J. A. Kremer Hovinga, B. Lämmle, H. J. Peter, and U. Schiemann. 2008. "Acute Pancreatitis and Thrombotic Thrombocytopenic Purpura." *European Journal of Medical Research* 13 (10): 481–82.

Bernardo, Aubrey, Chalmette Ball, Leticia Nolasco, Joel F. Moake, and Jing-fei Dong. 2004. "Effects of Inflammatory Cytokines on the Release and Cleavage of the Endothelial Cell-Derived Ultralarge von Willebrand Factor Multimers under Flow." *Blood* 104 (1): 100–106. https://doi.org/10.1182/blood-2004-01-0107.

Booth, Kristina K., Deirdra R. Terrell, Sara K. Vesely, and James N. George. 2011. "Systemic Infections Mimicking Thrombotic Thrombocytopenic Purpura." *American Journal of Hematology* 86 (9): 743–51. https://doi.org/10.1002/ajh.22091.

Brecher, Mark E., Shauna N. Hay, and Yara A. Park. 2008. "Is It HIV TTP or HIV-Associated Thrombotic Microangiopathy?" *Journal of Clinical Apheresis* 23 (6): 186–90. https://doi.org/10.1002/jca.20176.

Brichacek, Michal, Peter Blake, and Raymond Kao. 2012. "Capnocytophaga Canimorsus Infection Presenting with Complete Splenic Infarction and Thrombotic Thrombocytopenic Purpura: A Case Report." *BMC Research Notes* 5 (December): 695. https://doi.org/10.1186/1756-0500-5-695.

Camilleri, R. S., H. Cohen, I. J. Mackie, M. Scully, R. D. Starke, J. T. B. Crawley, D. A. Lane, and S. J. Machin. 2008. "Prevalence of the ADAMTS-13 Missense Mutation R1060W in Late Onset Adult Thrombotic Thrombocytopenic Purpura." *Journal of Thrombosis and Haemostasis: JTH* 6 (2): 331–38. https://doi.org/10.1111/j.1538-7836.2007.02846.x.

Chang, Jae C. 2018. "TTP-like Syndrome: Novel Concept and Molecular Pathogenesis of Endotheliopathy-Associated Vascular Microthrombotic Disease." *Thrombosis Journal* 16: 20. https://doi.org/10.1186/s12959-018-0174-4.

Chauhan, Anil K. 2014. "Degradation of Platelet-von Willebrand Factor Complexes by Plasmin: An Alternative/Backup Mechanism to ADAMTS13." *Circulation* 129 (12): 1273–75. https://doi.org/10.1161/CIRCULATIONAHA.114.008298.

Chitnis, Saurabh D., Tuoyo O. Mene-Afejuku, Amandeep Aujla, Ahmed Shady, Gaby S. Gil, Eder Hans Cativo, and Andrea Popescu-Martinez. 2017. "Thrombotic Thrombocytopenic Purpura Possibly Triggered by Graves' Disease." *Oxford Medical Case Reports* 2017 (10): omx057. https://doi.org/10.1093/omcr/omx057.

Coppo, P., M. Busson, A. Veyradier, A. Wynckel, P. Poullin, E. Azoulay, L. Galicier, P. Loiseau, and French Reference Centre For Thrombotic Microangiopathies. 2010. "HLA-DRB1*11: A Strong Risk Factor for Acquired Severe ADAMTS13 Deficiency-Related Idiopathic Thrombotic Thrombocytopenic Purpura in Caucasians." *Journal of Thrombosis and Haemostasis: JTH* 8 (4): 856–59. https://doi.org/10.1111/j.1538-7836.2010.03772.x.

De Cock, E., C. Hermans, J. De Raeymaecker, K. De Ceunynck, B. De Maeyer, N. Vandeputte, A. Vandenbulcke, et al. 2015. "The Novel ADAMTS13-p.D187H Mutation Impairs ADAMTS13 Activity and

Secretion and Contributes to Thrombotic Thrombocytopenic Purpura in Mice." *Journal of Thrombosis and Haemostasis: JTH* 13 (2): 283–92. https://doi.org/10.1111/jth.12804.

Du, Vivian X., Gwen van Os, Johanna A. Kremer Hovinga, Ilze Dienava-Verdoold, Jacques Wollersheim, Zaverio M. Ruggeri, Rob Fijnheer, Philip G. de Groot, and Bas de Laat. 2012. "Indications for a Protective Function of beta2-Glycoprotein I in Thrombotic Thrombocytopenic Purpura." *British Journal of Haematology* 159 (1): 94–103. https://doi.org/10.1111/bjh.12004.

Fox, Lucy C., Solomon J. Cohney, Joshua Y. Kausman, Jake Shortt, Peter D. Hughes, Erica M. Wood, Nicole M. Isbel, et al. 2018. "Consensus Opinion on Diagnosis and Management of Thrombotic Microangiopathy in Australia and New Zealand." *Nephrology (Carlton, Vic.)* 23 (6): 507–17. https://doi.org/10.1111/nep.13234.

Fujimura, Y., M. Matsumoto, A. Isonishi, H. Yagi, K. Kokame, K. Soejima, M. Murata, and T. Miyata. 2011. "Natural History of Upshaw-Schulman Syndrome Based on ADAMTS13 Gene Analysis in Japan." *Journal of Thrombosis and Haemostasis: JTH* 9 Suppl 1 (July): 283–301. https://doi.org/10.1111/j.1538-7836.2011.04341.x.

Fujimura, Yoshihiro, Masanori Matsumoto, Koichi Kokame, Ayami Isonishi, Kenji Soejima, Nobu Akiyama, Junji Tomiyama, et al. 2009. "Pregnancy-Induced Thrombocytopenia and TTP, and the Risk of Fetal Death, in Upshaw-Schulman Syndrome: A Series of 15 Pregnancies in 9 Genotyped Patients." *British Journal of Haematology* 144 (5): 742–54. https://doi.org/10.1111/j.1365-2141.2008.07515.x.

Furlan, M. 2000. "Von Willebrand Factor-Cleaving Protease in Thrombotic Thrombocytopenic Purpura and Hemolytic-Uremic Syndrome." *Advances in Nephrology from the Necker Hospital* 30: 71–81.

Furlan, M., and B. Lämmle. 2001. "Aetiology and Pathogenesis of Thrombotic Thrombocytopenic Purpura and Haemolytic Uraemic Syndrome: The Role of von Willebrand Factor-Cleaving Protease." *Best Practice & Research. Clinical Haematology* 14 (2): 437–54. https://doi.org/10.1053/beha.2001.0142.

Furlan, M., R. Robles, B. Morselli, P. Sandoz, and B. Lämmle. 1999. "Recovery and Half-Life of von Willebrand Factor-Cleaving Protease after Plasma Therapy in Patients with Thrombotic Thrombocytopenic Purpura." *Thrombosis and Haemostasis* 81 (1): 8–13.

George, James N. 2003. "The Association of Pregnancy with Thrombotic Thrombocytopenic Purpura-Hemolytic Uremic Syndrome." *Current Opinion in Hematology* 10 (5): 339–44.

———. 2011. "Systemic Malignancies as a Cause of Unexpected Microangiopathic Hemolytic Anemia and Thrombocytopenia." *Oncology (Williston Park, N.Y.)* 25 (10): 908–14.

George, James N., Sara K. Vesely, and Judith A. James. 2007. "Overlapping Features of Thrombotic Thrombocytopenic Purpura and Systemic Lupus Erythematosus." *Southern Medical Journal* 100 (5): 512–14. https://doi.org/10.1097/SMJ.0b013e318046583f.

George JM, Cuker A. 2018a. *Acquired TTP: Clinical Manifestations and Diagnosis.* UpToDate.

———. 2018b. *Hereditary Thrombotic Thrombocytopenic Purpura (TTP).* UpToDate.

———. 2018c. *Pathophysiology of Acquired TTP and Other Primary Thrombotic Microangiopathies (TMAs).* UpToDate.

Hamasaki, K., T. Mimura, H. Kanda, K. Kubo, K. Setoguchi, T. Satoh, Y. Misaki, and K. Yamamoto. 2003. "Systemic Lupus Erythematosus and Thrombotic Thrombocytopenic Purpura: A Case Report and Literature Review." *Clinical Rheumatology* 22 (4–5): 355–58. https://doi.org/10.1007/s10067-003-0742-1.

Hanby, Hayley A., and X. Long Zheng. 2014. "Current Status in Diagnosis and Treatment of Hereditary Thrombotic Thrombocytopenic Purpura." *Hereditary Genetics: Current Research* 3 (1). https://doi.org/10.4172/2161-1041.1000e108.

Jiang, Yang, Jennifer J. McIntosh, Jessica A. Reese, Cassandra C. Deford, Johanna A. Kremer Hovinga, Bernhard Lämmle, Deirdra R. Terrell, Sara K. Vesely, Eric J. Knudtson, and James N. George. 2014. "Pregnancy Outcomes Following Recovery from Acquired Thrombotic

Thrombocytopenic Purpura." *Blood* 123 (11): 1674–80. https://doi.org/10.1182/blood-2013-11-538900.

John, Marie-Luise, Walter Hitzler, and Inge Scharrer. 2012. "The Role of Human Leukocyte Antigens as Predisposing And/Or Protective Factors in Patients with Idiopathic Thrombotic Thrombocytopenic Purpura." *Annals of Hematology* 91 (4): 507–10. https://doi.org/10.1007/s00277-011-1384-z.

Joly, Bérangère S., Alain Stepanian, Thierry Leblanc, David Hajage, Hervé Chambost, Jérôme Harambat, Fanny Fouyssac, et al. 2016. "Child-Onset and Adolescent-Onset Acquired Thrombotic Thrombocytopenic Purpura with Severe ADAMTS13 Deficiency: A Cohort Study of the French National Registry for Thrombotic Microangiopathy." *The Lancet. Haematology* 3 (11): e537–46. https://doi.org/10.1016/S2352-3026(16)30125-9.

Joseph, A. and Fangio P. 2015. "Seasonal Flu as a Triggering Factor for Acquired Thrombotic Thrombocytopenic Purpura." *Journal of Hematology & Thromboembolic Diseases* 4 (3). https://doi.org/10.4172/2329-8790.1000243.

Kentouche, K., A. Voigt, E. Schleussner, R. Schneppenheim, U. Budde, J. F. Beck, E. Stefańska-Windyga, and J. Windyga. 2013. "Pregnancy in Upshaw-Schulman Syndrome." *Hamostaseologie* 33 (2): 144–48. https://doi.org/10.5482/HAMO-13-04-0025.

Kosugi, Nobuharu, Yuya Tsurutani, Ayami Isonishi, Yuji Hori, Masanori Matsumoto, and Yoshihiro Fujimura. 2010. "Influenza A Infection Triggers Thrombotic Thrombocytopenic Purpura by Producing the Anti-ADAMTS13 IgG Inhibitor." *Internal Medicine (Tokyo, Japan)* 49 (7): 689–93.

Kremer Hovinga, Johanna A., Paul Coppo, Bernhard Lämmle, Joel L. Moake, Toshiyuki Miyata, and Karen Vanhoorelbeke. 2017. "Thrombotic Thrombocytopenic Purpura." *Nature Reviews. Disease Primers* 3 (April): 17020. https://doi.org/10.1038/nrdp.2017.20.

Krogh, A. S. von, P. Quist-Paulsen, A. Waage, Ø O. Langseth, K. Thorstensen, R. Brudevold, G. E. Tjønnfjord, C. R. Largiadèr, B. Lämmle, and J. A. Kremer Hovinga. 2016. "High Prevalence of

Hereditary Thrombotic Thrombocytopenic Purpura in Central Norway: From Clinical Observation to Evidence." *Journal of Thrombosis and Haemostasis: JTH* 14 (1): 73–82. https://doi.org/10.1111/jth.13186.

Levy, G. G., W. C. Nichols, E. C. Lian, T. Foroud, J. N. McClintick, B. M. McGee, A. Y. Yang, et al. 2001. "Mutations in a Member of the ADAMTS Gene Family Cause Thrombotic Thrombocytopenic Purpura." *Nature* 413 (6855): 488–94. https://doi.org/10.1038/35097008.

Liu, L., H. Choi, A. Bernardo, A. L. Bergeron, L. Nolasco, C. Ruan, J. L. Moake, and J.-F. Dong. 2005. "Platelet-Derived VWF-Cleaving Metalloprotease ADAMTS-13." *Journal of Thrombosis and Haemostasis: JTH* 3 (11): 2536–44. https://doi.org/10.1111/j.1538-7836.2005.01561.x.

Lopes da Silva, Rodrigo. 2011. "Viral-Associated Thrombotic Microangiopathies." *Hematology/Oncology and Stem Cell Therapy* 4 (2): 51–59.

Mal, Hervé, Agnès Veyradier, Olivier Brugière, Daniel Da Silva, Magali Colombat, Elie Azoulay, Laurent Benayoun, et al. 2006. "Thrombotic Microangiopathy with Acquired Deficiency in ADAMTS 13 Activity in Lung Transplant Recipients." *Transplantation* 81 (12): 1628–32. https://doi.org/10.1097/01.tp.0000226066.82066.fa.

Manea, Minola, Ramesh Tati, Jessica Karlsson, Zivile D. Békássy, and Diana Karpman. 2010. "Biologically Active ADAMTS13 Is Expressed in Renal Tubular Epithelial Cells." *Pediatric Nephrology (Berlin, Germany)* 25 (1): 87–96. https://doi.org/10.1007/s00467-009-1262-2.

Martino, Suella, Mathieu Jamme, Christophe Deligny, Marc Busson, Pascale Loiseau, Elie Azoulay, Lionel Galicier, et al. 2016. "Thrombotic Thrombocytopenic Purpura in Black People: Impact of Ethnicity on Survival and Genetic Risk Factors." *PloS One* 11 (7): e0156679. https://doi.org/10.1371/journal.pone.0156679.

Mead, Timothy J., and Suneel S. Apte. 2018. "ADAMTS Proteins in Human Disorders." *Matrix Biology: Journal of the International Society for Matrix Biology* 71–72 (October): 225–39. https://doi.org/10.1016/j.matbio.2018.06.002.

Meyer, S. C. et al. 2007. "The ADAMTS13 Gene as the Immunological Culprit in Acute Acquired TTP — First Evidence of Genetic out-Breeding Depression in Humans." *Blood* 110: 277.

Miner, Paul F., Robert L. Nutt, and Miles E. Thomas. 1955. "Thrombotic Thrombocytopenic Purpura Occurring in Pregnancy." *American Journal of Obstetrics and Gynecology* 70 (3): 611–17. https://doi.org/10.1016/0002-9378(55)90355-0.

Miyata, T., K. Kokame, M. Matsumoto, and Y. Fujimura. 2013. "ADAMTS13 Activity and Genetic Mutations in Japan." *Hamostaseologie* 33 (2): 131–37. https://doi.org/10.5482/HAMO-12-11-0017.

Moake, J. L., C. K. Rudy, J. H. Troll, M. J. Weinstein, N. M. Colannino, J. Azocar, R. H. Seder, S. L. Hong, and D. Deykin. 1982. "Unusually Large Plasma Factor VIII: von Willebrand Factor Multimers in Chronic Relapsing Thrombotic Thrombocytopenic Purpura." *The New England Journal of Medicine* 307 (23): 1432–35. https://doi.org/10.1056/NEJM198212023072306.

Moatti-Cohen, M., C. Garrec, M. Wolf, P. Boisseau, L. Galicier, E. Azoulay, A. Stepanian, et al. 2012. "Unexpected Frequency of Upshaw-Schulman Syndrome in Pregnancy-Onset Thrombotic Thrombocytopenic Purpura." *Blood* 119 (24): 5888–97. https://doi.org/10.1182/blood-2012-02-408914.

Morton, Jordan M., and James N. George. 2016. "Microangiopathic Hemolytic Anemia and Thrombocytopenia in Patients With Cancer." *Journal of Oncology Practice* 12 (6): 523–30. https://doi.org/10.1200/JOP.2016.012096.

Moschcowitz, Eli. 1925. "An acute febrile pleiochromic anemia with hyaline thrombosis of the terminal arterioles and capillaries: An undescribed disease." *Archives of Internal Medicine* 36 (1): 89. https://doi.org/10.1001/archinte.1925.00120130092009.

Opie, Jessica. 2012. "Haematological Complications of HIV Infection." *South African Medical Journal = Suid-Afrikaanse Tydskrif Vir Geneeskunde* 102 (6): 465–68.

Page, E. E., J. A. Kremer Hovinga, D. R. Terrell, S. K. Vesely, and J. N. George. 2016. "Clinical Importance of ADAMTS13 Activity during Remission in Patients with Acquired Thrombotic Thrombocytopenic Purpura." *Blood* 128 (17): 2175–78. https://doi.org/10.1182/blood-2016-06-724161.

Pillai, Vikram G., Jialing Bao, Catherine B. Zander, Jenny K. McDaniel, Palaniappan S. Chetty, Steven H. Seeholzer, Khalil Bdeir, Douglas B. Cines, and X. Long Zheng. 2016. "Human Neutrophil Peptides Inhibit Cleavage of von Willebrand Factor by ADAMTS13: A Potential Link of Inflammation to TTP." *Blood* 128 (1): 110–19. https://doi.org/10.1182/blood-2015-12-688747.

Reese, Jessica A., Daniel W. Bougie, Brian R. Curtis, Deirdra R. Terrell, Sara K. Vesely, Richard H. Aster, and James N. George. 2015. "Drug-Induced Thrombotic Microangiopathy: Experience of the Oklahoma Registry and the BloodCenter of Wisconsin." *American Journal of Hematology* 90 (5): 406–10. https://doi.org/10.1002/ajh.23960.

Reese, Jessica A., Darrshini S. Muthurajah, Johanna A. Kremer Hovinga, Sara K. Vesely, Deirdra R. Terrell, and James N. George. 2013. "Children and Adults with Thrombotic Thrombocytopenic Purpura Associated with Severe, Acquired Adamts13 Deficiency: Comparison of Incidence, Demographic and Clinical Features." *Pediatric Blood & Cancer* 60 (10): 1676–82. https://doi.org/10.1002/pbc.24612.

Registry Hereditary Thrombotic thrombo-citopenic purpura/Upshaw Schulman syndrome. ClinicalTrial.gov identifier: NCT01257269. Accessed December 2018. http://www.ttpregistry.net

Sadler, J. Evan. 2017. "Pathophysiology of Thrombotic Thrombocytopenic Purpura." *Blood* 130 (10): 1181–88. https://doi.org/10.1182/blood-2017-04-636431.

Saha, M., J. K. McDaniel, and X. L. Zheng. 2017. "Thrombotic Thrombocytopenic Purpura: Pathogenesis, Diagnosis and Potential Novel Therapeutics." *Journal of Thrombosis and Haemostasis* 15 (10): 1889–1900. https://doi.org/10.1111/jth.13764.

Sayarlioglu, Mehmet, Hayriye Sayarlioglu, Mesut Ozkaya, Ozan Balakan, and Mehmet Ali Ucar. 2008. "Thrombotic Thrombocytopenic Purpura-

Hemolytic Uremic Syndrome and Adult Onset Still's Disease: Case Report and Review of the Literature." *Modern Rheumatology* 18 (4): 403–6. https://doi.org/10.1007/s10165-008-0061-0.

Schneppenheim, Reinhard, Johanna A. Kremer Hovinga, Tim Becker, Ulrich Budde, Diana Karpman, Wolfgang Brockhaus, Ingrid Hrachovinová, et al. 2006. "A Common Origin of the 4143insA ADAMTS13 Mutation." *Thrombosis and Haemostasis* 96 (1): 3–6. https://doi.org/10.1160/TH05-12-0817.

Schulman, I., M. Pierce, A. Lukens, and Z. Currimbhoy. 1960. "Studies on Thrombopoiesis. I. A Factor in Normal Human Plasma Required for Platelet Production; Chronic Thrombocytopenia due to Its Deficiency." *Blood* 16 (July): 943–57.

Scully, M., M. Thomas, M. Underwood, H. Watson, K. Langley, R. S. Camilleri, A. Clark, et al. 2014. "Thrombotic Thrombocytopenic Purpura and Pregnancy: Presentation, Management, and Subsequent Pregnancy Outcomes." *Blood* 124 (2): 211–19. https://doi.org/10.1182/blood-2014-02-553131.

Scully, Marie, Beverley J. Hunt, Sylvia Benjamin, Ri Liesner, Peter Rose, Flora Peyvandi, Betty Cheung, Samuel J. Machin, and British Committee for Standards in Haematology. 2012. "Guidelines on the Diagnosis and Management of Thrombotic Thrombocytopenic Purpura and Other Thrombotic Microangiopathies." *British Journal of Haematology* 158 (3): 323–35. https://doi.org/10.1111/j.1365-2141.2012.09167.x.

Scully, Marie, Helen Yarranton, Ri Liesner, Jamie Cavenagh, Beverley Hunt, Sylvia Benjamin, David Bevan, Ian Mackie, and Samuel Machin. 2008. "Regional UK TTP Registry: Correlation with Laboratory ADAMTS 13 Analysis and Clinical Features." *British Journal of Haematology* 142 (5): 819–26. https://doi.org/10.1111/j.1365-2141.2008.07276.x.

Shelat, Suresh G., Jihui Ai, and X. Long Zheng. 2005. "Molecular Biology of ADAMTS13 and Diagnostic Utility of ADAMTS13 Proteolytic Activity and Inhibitor Assays." *Seminars in Thrombosis and Hemostasis* 31 (6): 659–72. https://doi.org/10.1055/s-2005-925472.

Smeets, Nori J. L., Rob Fijnheer, Silvie Sebastian, and Quirijn De Mast. 2018. "Secondary Thrombotic Microangiopathy with Severely Reduced ADAMTS13 Activity in a Patient with Capnocytophaga Canimorsus Sepsis: A Case Report." *Transfusion* 58 (10): 2426–29. https://doi.org/10.1111/trf.14829.

Suzuki, Eiji, Takashi Kanno, Tomoyuki Asano, Akito Tsutsumi, Hiroko Kobayashi, Hiroshi Watanabe, and Hiromasa Ohira. 2013. "Two Cases of Mixed Connective Tissue Disease Complicated with Thrombotic Thrombocytopenic Purpura." *Fukushima Journal of Medical Science* 59 (1): 49–55.

Taleghani, M., A.-S. von Krogh, Y. Fujimura, J. N. George, I. Hrachovinova, P. N. Knöbl, P. Quist-Paulsen, R. Schneppenheim, B. Lämmle, and J. A. Hovinga. 2013. "Hereditary thrombotic thrombocytopenic purpura and the hereditary TTP registry." *Hämostaseologie* 33 (2): 138–43. https://doi.org/10.5482/HAMO-13-04-0026.

Terrell, D. R., L. A. Williams, S. K. Vesely, B. Lämmle, J. a. K. Hovinga, and J. N. George. 2005. "The Incidence of Thrombotic Thrombocytopenic Purpura-Hemolytic Uremic Syndrome: All Patients, Idiopathic Patients, and Patients with Severe ADAMTS-13 Deficiency." *Journal of Thrombosis and Haemostasis: JTH* 3 (7): 1432–36. https://doi.org/10.1111/j.1538-7836.2005.01436.x.

Tersteeg, Claudia, Steven de Maat, Simon F. De Meyer, Michel W. J. Smeets, Arjan D. Barendrecht, Mark Roest, Gerard Pasterkamp, et al. 2014. "Plasmin Cleavage of von Willebrand Factor as an Emergency Bypass for ADAMTS13 Deficiency in Thrombotic Microangiopathy." *Circulation* 129 (12): 1320–31. https://doi.org/10.1161/CIRCULATION AHA.113.006727.

Tsai, H. M., and E. C. Lian. 1998. "Antibodies to von Willebrand Factor-Cleaving Protease in Acute Thrombotic Thrombocytopenic Purpura." *The New England Journal of Medicine* 339 (22): 1585–94. https://doi.org/10.1056/NEJM199811263392203.

Tsai, H. M., L. Rice, R. Sarode, T. W. Chow, and J. L. Moake. 2000. "Antibody Inhibitors to von Willebrand Factor Metalloproteinase and

Increased Binding of von Willebrand Factor to Platelets in Ticlopidine-Associated Thrombotic Thrombocytopenic Purpura." *Annals of Internal Medicine* 132 (10): 794–99.

Turner, N., L. Nolasco, Z. Tao, J.-F. Dong, and J. Moake. 2006. "Human Endothelial Cells Synthesize and Release ADAMTS-13." *Journal of Thrombosis and Haemostasis: JTH* 4 (6): 1396–1404. https://doi.org/10.1111/j.1538-7836.2006.01959.x.

Upshaw, J. D. 1978. "Congenital Deficiency of a Factor in Normal Plasma That Reverses Microangiopathic Hemolysis and Thrombocytopenia." *The New England Journal of Medicine* 298 (24): 1350–52. https://doi.org/10.1056/NEJM197806152982407.

Verweij, C. L., P. J. Diergaarde, M. Hart, and H. Pannekoek. 1986. "Full-Length von Willebrand Factor (vWF) cDNA Encodes a Highly Repetitive Protein Considerably Larger than the Mature vWF Subunit." *The EMBO Journal* 5 (8): 1839–47.

Xu, Xiaohan, Tienan Zhu, Di Wu, and Lu Zhang. 2018. "Sjögren's Syndrome Initially Presented as Thrombotic Thrombocytopenic Purpura in a Male Patient: A Case Report and Literature Review." *Clinical Rheumatology* 37 (5): 1421–26. https://doi.org/10.1007/s10067-017-3912-2.

Yamashita, Hiroyuki, Yuko Takahashi, Hiroshi Kaneko, Toshikazu Kano, and Akio Mimori. 2013. "Thrombotic Thrombocytopenic Purpura with an Autoantibody to ADAMTS13 Complicating Sjögren's Syndrome: Two Cases and a Literature Review." *Modern Rheumatology* 23 (2): 365–73. https://doi.org/10.1007/s10165-012-0644-7.

Zander, Catherine B., Wenjing Cao, and X. Long Zheng. 2015. "ADAMTS13 and von Willebrand Factor Interactions." *Current Opinion in Hematology* 22 (5): 452–59. https://doi.org/10.1097/MOH.0000000000000169.

Zheng, Xinglong, Elaine M. Majerus, and J. Evan Sadler. 2002. "ADAMTS13 and TTP." *Current Opinion in Hematology* 9 (5): 389–94.

In: Thrombotic Thrombocytopenic Purpura ISBN: 978-1-53615-353-8
Editor: Mason Hillam © 2019 Nova Science Publishers, Inc.

Chapter 2

DIAGNOSIS OF THROMBOTIC THROMBOCYTOPENIC PURPURA

Ana Dolores Del Rey Luján[1,*], MD,
Carmen Cristina Amorós Pérez[2], MD,
Llanos Belmonte Andújar[3], MD, Lorena Pico Rico[1], MD
and Martin Antonio Cabero Becerra[1], MD

[1]Hematology and Hemotherapy
Hospital of Alcázar de San Juan, Ciudad Real, Spain
[2]Hematology and Hemotherapy,
Hospital Virgen de los Lirios, Alcoy, Alicante, Spain
[3]Obstetrics and Gynecology Department,
Hospital of Almansa, Albacete, Spain

---

[*] Correspondence Author's E- mail: anadelrey22@hotmail.com.

ABSTRACT

Thrombotic thrombocytopenic purpura (TTP) is a rare and life-threatening thrombotic microangiopathy characterized by microangiopathic hemolytic anemia, severe thrombocytopenia, and organ ischemia related to disseminated thrombosis. In 1924, TTP was first clinically described by Eli Moschcowitz in a 16-year-old girl as fatal thrombotic microangiopathy. Until the 1980s to 1990s, the etiology for TTP remained unknown. During the last few years, different hypotheses have been considered, including genetic alterations that could cause a predisposition to PTT, the most common: ADAMTS 13 mutations.

TTP is twice as frequent in women, and its outcome is characterized by being prone to relapse. Rapid recognition of TTP is crucial to initiate appropriate treatment, without treatment, it leads to death in 90% of patients, often during the first 24 hours, mainly due to ischemic episodes.

The incidence of acquired PTT is much higher in adults (2.9 cases /million/year) than in children (0.1 cases/ million/year). Acquired thrombotic thrombocytopenic purpura usually presents with an acute clinical course, with a tendency to relapse and occasional association of other autoimmune disorders. The classic clinical description of PTT has been the pentad of microangiopathic hemolytic anemia, thrombocytopenia, fever, renal failure and neurologic findings, but not all patients present it.

The diagnosis of PTT is made by standard laboratory tests: In addition to the microangiopathic hemolytic anemia and consumption thrombocytopenia, classical parameters for hemolysis show an elevated reticulocyte count, an undetectable serum haptoglobin concentration, and a markedly elevated lactate dehydrogenase level as well as the presence of schistocytes on the blood smear. Direct antiglobulin (Coombs) test (DAT) is negative. Standard coagulation parameters are usually normal, but severe organ ischemia may cause disseminated intravascular coagulation, which is associated with coagulation abnormalities. Kidney assessment may show proteinuria, hematuria, and sometimes elevated plasma urea and creatinine levels.

As these standard investigations are not specific for TTP, they must be accompanied by the assessment of ADAMTS13, the unique sensitive and specific marker for TTP. The specialized laboratories can determine 3 aspects related to ADAMTS13: antigen, activity and presence of antibodies. The ADAMTS13 activity is the main parameter to be evaluated due to its informative value regarding the functionality of the molecule.

INTRODUCTION

Thrombotic microangiopathy (TMA) refers to a pathologic lesion seen on tissue biopsy; however, the presence of a TMA is often inferred from clinical features such as microangiopathic hemolytic anemia (MAHA) and thrombocytopenia, along with signs of organ injury. Primary TMA refers to a TMA for which a specific cause requires specific management. Examples include acquired TTP, hereditary TTP, Shiga toxin-mediated hemolytic uremic syndrome (ST-HUS), complement-mediated HUS, drug-induced TMA, and other rare inherited TMA syndromes.

TTP was first described in 1924 by Moschowitz as a disease presenting with a pentad of signs and symptoms (anemia, thrombocytopenia, fever, hemiparesis and hematuria) (Moschcowitz E. 1924). Because fever, neurological and renal involvement is not constant in patients, especially in early forms of the disease, the definition changed to a non-immune microangiopathic hemolytic anemia with erythrocyte fragmentation and consumption thrombocytopenia, in the absence of alternative causes that explain these findings.

The description of von Willebrand factor (VWF) multimers of unusually large size in the plasma of patients with TTP represented a turning point for the understanding of the disease pathophysiology (Moake JL, Rudy CK, Troll JH, Weinstein MJ, Colannino NM, Azocar J, et al. 1982) (Moake JL. 2002). The presence in plasma of the highly platelet-adhesive unusually large multimers of VWF provided a plausible explanation for the platelet- and VWF-rich thrombi observed in the small vessels of patients with TTP. Studies in the late 1990s then independently demonstrated the severe deficiency of a specific VWF cleaving-protease in the plasma of patients with recurrent TTP (Furlan M, Robles R, Solenthaler M, Wassmer M, Sandoz P, Lammle B 1997). This protease was identified as the thirteenth member of the ADAMTS family of metalloproteases, ADAMTS13 (Gerritsen HE, Robles R, Lammle B, Furlan M 2001)(Fujikawa K, Suzuki H, McMullen B, Chung D. 2001)(Zheng X, Chung D, Takayama TK, Majerus EM, Sadler JE, Fujikawa K 2001).

There are two types de TTP: The congenital form or Upshaw-Schulman syndrome is an autosomal recessive disorder and the acquired form can be idiopathic or occur in the context of cancer, autoimmune diseases or drug administration (example: cyclosporine, quinine, etc.). When it occurs during pregnancy, it can be confused with severe pre-eclampsia.

Hereditary TTP represents less than 5% of all TTP cases; over 95% are acquired autoimmune TTP. However, among certain groups such as newborn infants and young children, hereditary TTP may be more common than acquired TTP. In pregnant women, hereditary TTP may represent up to one-fourth of TTP cases (Moatti-Cohen M, Garrec C, Wolf M, et al. 2012).

The overall mortality of TTP used to be higher than 90%, but it has decreased to 8–30% after the introduction of plasma exchange therapy, which is the treatment of choice of acute TTP episodes. 17-20 Up to 40% of patients with TTP develop recurrent episodes of the disease, with the risk of recurrences being higher in patients with severe ADAMTS13 deficiency and anti-ADAMTS13 autoanti-bodies during acute episodes (Zheng XL, Kaufman RM, Goodnough LT, Sadler JE 2004) (Hovinga JA, Vesely SK, Terrell DR, Lammle B, George JN 2010) (Vesely SK, George JN, Lämmle B, Studt JD, Alberio L, El-Harake MA, et al. 2003) (Raife T, Atkinson B, Montgomery R, Vesely S, Friedman K. 2004) (Coppo P, Bengoufa D, Veyradier A, Wolf M, Bussel A, Millot GA, et al. 2004).

CLASSIFICATION AND EPIDEMIOLOGY

There are two types of TTP:

- Congenital TTP (Upshaw-Schulman syndrome):
  o The incidence of hereditary TTP appears to be a very rare disorder. In the Oklahoma TTP-HUS Registry (which includes any patient referred for clinical suspicion of TTP or hemolytic uremic syndrome), representing a population base of 2 million people. A population-based cross sectional study in Norway discovered an unexpectedly high prevalence, with 17

individuals affected per one million population (Von Krogh AS, Quist-Paulsen P, Waage A, et al. 2016).
- o It is caused by homozygous or compound heterozygous mutations in the ADAMTS13 gene. So far, more than 150 mutations of ADAMTS13 have been described, which include missense mutations (approximately 60%), small deletions and insertions (approximately 20%), as well as nonsense and mutations of the splice site, although studies of expression have been carried out only for some of them (Lotta LA, Garagiola I, Palla R, Cairo A, Peyvandi F 2010) (Calderazzo JC, Kempfer A, Powazniak Y, López IR, Sánchez-Luceros A, Woods AI, Lazzari MA 2012).
- Acquired TTP.
- o The incidence of idiopathic TTP is estimated to be 4.5/1 million person/year, being higher in people of black ethnicity, based on data from the Oklahoma TTP-HUS Registry (Reese JA, Muthurajah DS, Kremer Hovinga JA, et al. 2013). The male to female ratio is 1:2, similar to the ratio for other autoimmune diseases. (Terrell DR, Williams LA, Vesely SK, Lämmle B, Hovinga JA, George JN. 2005). The median age for the diagnosis of acquired TTP is 41, with a wide range (9 to 78 years). It is very rare in children, the incidence in children <18 years old is approximately 1 per 10 million per year (Reese JA, Muthurajah DS, Kremer Hovinga JA, et al. 2013).
- o It is caused by the production of anti-ADAMTS13 auto-antibodies. Depending on its origin, acquired TTP may be:
    - Idiopatic: when the cause of TTP is ignored and there is no known underlying or associated condition.
    - Secondary: when the development of TTP is due to a predisposing or precipitating factor.

CLINICAL PRESENTATION

Patients with hereditary TTP have similar presenting symptoms as those with acquired TTP during an acute episode, but hereditary TTP often presents during the neonatal or childhood period. Among adults, presentation during pregnancy is common.

Patients with TTP present with a wide range of symptoms, not immediately suspicious for TTP, such as abdominal pain, nausea and vomiting. There are theories that postulate that some of these symptoms reflect an underlying disease that may have triggered TTP (Kosugi N, Tsurutani Y, Isonishi A, Hori Y, Matusmoto M, Fujimura Y. 2010). Unfortunately, the nonspecific nature of signs and symptoms of TTP are likely to hamper a physician's ability to suspect it on clinical grounds alone. Unless a complete blood cell count is ordered and the combination of severe thrombocytopenia and microangiopathic hemolytic anemia is noted, it is concerning that some patients may experience a delay in diagnosis.

Anecdotally, we know that many patients are seen by several physicians until the constellation of history, laboratory results and consultation with colleagues in hematology or apheresis medicine eventually leads to the correct diagnosis of TTP.

Symptoms

1. Neurologic: Incidence 52-92%. Neurologic findings are common; especially subtle changes such as confusion and headache (Page EE, Kremer Hovinga JA, Terrell DR, et al. 2017) (George JN. 2010) (George JN. 2006) (Sadler JE, Moake JL, Miyata T, George JN. 2017)(George JN. 2017). Transient focal neurologic findings such as difficulty speaking or transient numbness and weakness, seizures, and coma also occur (Scully M, Yarranton H, Liesner R, et al. 2014). In a series of 78 patients with TTP, minor abnormalities such as confusion or headache were seen in 21 (27%); focal abnormalities were seen in 31 (40%); and fewer patients had seizure, stroke or

coma (15, 12 and 8 percent, respectively) (Page EE, Kremer Hovinga JA, Terrell DR, et al. 2017).
2. Gastrointestinal: Variable incidence. Gastrointestinal symptoms are common and may include pain, nausea, vomiting or diarrhea. In one series of 65 patients with TTP, these gastrointestinal symptoms were the most common finding, seen in 45 individuals (69%). It is important to establish the timeframe between diarrhea and other TMA symptoms, if possible. In Shiga toxin-induced TMA a prodromal gastrointestinal illness with abdominal pain, vomiting, and diarrhea generally precedes the development of MAHA and thrombocytopenia by several days (Page EE, Kremer Hovinga JA, Terrell DR, et al. 2017).
3. Renal Insufficiency: Incidence 76-88%. Renal insufficiency can be seen in TTP, but anuria and acute renal failure are rare (Page EE, Kremer Hovinga JA, Terrell DR, et al. 2017) (George JN, Nester CM 2014). In the Oklahoma series of patients with TTP, the median serum creatinine was 1,3mg/dL (115micromol/L) (Page EE, Kremer Hovinga JA, Terrell DR, et al. 2017). Of 78 patients, 37 had normal renal function (47,5%), 37 had increased serum creatinine (47,5%), and four had acute renal failure (5%), which was defined as an increasing serum creatinine (> 0,5mg/dL per day for two consecutive days) or a serum creatinine >4mg/dL and hemodialysis. 23. Of note, a separate study suggested that acute kidney injury may be common in patients with TTP who are hospitalized in a referral center intensive care unit (Zafrani L, Mariotte E, Darmon M, et al. 2015). The urinalysis is normal or may show mild proteinuria (e.g., 1 to 2 g per day) and few cells or cast (Remuzzi G. 1987) (Remuzzi G 1986). These findings of mild or no renal insufficiency contrast with other primary TMA syndromes such as Shiga toxin-associated hemolytic uremic syndrome, complement-mediated TMA, or immune mediated drug-induced TMA (e.g., due to quinine), in which acute kidney injury with anuria may be common.
4. Cardiac: Variable incidence. Cardiac involvement may occur in TTP, although the exact incidence may be difficult to determine. In

one series of 65 patients with TTP, 14 had chest pain (22%). Other series have reported arrhythmia, sudden cardiac death, myocardial infarction, cardiogenic shock, and/or heart failure (Hawkins BM, Abu-Fadel M, Vesely SK, George JN. 2008) (Gami AS, Hayman SR, Grande JP, Garovic VD. 2005) (Patschan D, Witzke O, Dührsen U, et al. 2006) (Hughes C, McEwan JR, Longair I, et al. 2009).
5. Fever. Incidence 24-98%. If the fever is high, rule out infectious process.
6. Asthenia. Variable incidence. It may be caused by haemolytic anemia.
7. Hemorrhage. Variable incidence. Bleeding from the gums or nose, which may be caused by thrombocytopenia. Purple bruises on the skin, called purpura, and red or purple maculae on the skin, called petechiae, which are caused by bleeding under the skin.
8. Dark urine from hemoglobinuria may be caused by haemolytic anemia.

Involvement of other organs, including pancreas, thyroid, adrenal glands, and other organs, may also be seen. Pulmonary involvement is rare (Nokes T, George JN, Vesely SK, Awab A. 2014).

LABORATORY FINDINGS

The initial evaluation is focused on confirming that the patient has true MAHA and thrombocytopenia, and excluding systemic disorders that manifest these findings, based on a consideration of presented findings and likely causes (George JN, Nester CM 2014). Once systemic disorders have been excluded, the focus changes to identifying which primary TMA syndromes are most likely and require immediate treatment.

Importantly, we favor starting with a thorough history and physical examination that guides selected use of laboratory tests rather than a battery of test to confirm or exclude a large number of diagnosis, especially as many available tests are not highly sensitive or specific for a single diagnosis.

Institutions may develop their own approaches depending on their case mix and associated likely diagnosis, but these should not substitute the judgment of the clinician evaluating the patient (Go RS, Winters JL, Leung N, et al. 2016).

Hemogram: MAHA and Thrombocytopenia

The possibility of TTP should be evaluated in any patient who presents with these findings without an apparent alternative explanation. Confirmation of both of these findings requires review of the peripheral blood smear by an experienced clinician. Automated instruments and less experienced individuals may mistake other red blood cell (RBC) abnormalities for microangiopathic changes (e.g., anisopoikilocytosis, megaloblastic changes, teardrop cell…) (Routh JK, Koenig SC. 2014) (Noël N, Maigné G, Tertian G, et al. 2013).

Microangiopathic Hemolytic Anemia (MAHA)

Incidence 100%. It is a hemolytic anemia that results from mechanical shearing (fragmentation) of RBC as they pass through platelet-rich microthrombi in the microvasculature; it is documented by the finding of prominent schistocytes, including helmet cell and triangular cells, on the peripheral blood smear (Brain MC, Dacie JV, Hourihane DO 1962). Polychromasia is common. Microspherocytes and nucleated RBCs may also be seen, but microspherocytes are more prominent in patients with warm autoimmune hemolytic anemia and many nucleated red cells may suggest a myelophistic process, such as metastatic malignancy, that may mimic the clinical features of TTP.

The abundance of schistocytes is variable in TTP and can be affected by the duration of disease and the quality of the blood smear preparation. A finding of two or more schistocytes per high power field (e.g., viewed by a 100X magnification oil immersion objective) in the appropriate clinical setting is suggestive of MAHA (George JN. 2010). The quantity of schistocytes in TTP was illustrated in a series of patients with TTP and other disorders typically associated with MAHA, in which schistocytes represented on average 8% of RBCs in the patients with TTP (Burns ER, Lou Y, Pathak A. 2004). This percentage was substantially higher than that seen in patients with other disorders associated with MAHA (e.g., scleroderma renal crisis and other severe kidney disorders, preeclampsia, mechanical heart valve), all of whom had < 0,5% schistocytes (Brain MC, Dacie JV, Hourihane DO 1962). Importantly, however, there is no threshold schistocyte number below which the possibility of TTP can be excluded.

The presence of one or two schistocytes in a single field has a very low specificity for TTP. However, more subtle signs of RBC fragmentation may be seen, especially early in disease presentation, and an early involvement of the consulting hematologist and/or hematopathologist is encouraged. Rarely, a patient with early TTP may not have schistocytes appreciated; this may occur in a patient in the early stages of relapse who is being followed closely (Fava S, Galizia AC. 1995).

Thrombocytopenia

Incidence 100%. It is thought to result from deposition of platelets in microthrombi, severe thrombocytopenia is common. This was illustrated in a series of 78 patients with TTP, in which the mean platelet count on presentation was 10.000/microL (Page EE, Kremer Hovinga JA, Terrell DR, et al. 2017). Bleeding is sometimes seen; it may result from a combination of thrombocytopenia, vascular injury and/or tissue infarction. In the same series, bleeding, typically petechiae and purpura, was reported in 35 of 65 patients (54%) (George JN. 2010). Major over bleeding is very rare.

It is important confirming thrombocytopenia on the peripheral blood smear (to exclude pseudothrombocytopenia).

Biochemistry

- Elevation of the serum indirect bilirubin concentration
- Reduction in the serum haptoglobin concentration.

- Reticulocyte count generally increased to compensate for accelerated red cell destruction.
- Serum lactate dehydrogenase level is typically extremely high, reflecting both hemolysis and tissue damage due to systemic ischemia.
- Coombs testing is negative.
- Coagulation: Plasma times and fibrinogen levels are almost always normal, but severe organ ischemia may cause disseminated intravascular coagulation, which is associated with coagulation abnormalities.

Additional Diagnostic Testing May Be Appropriate in Selected Patients

- Imaging: Computed tomography or magnetic resonance imaging of the brain may be appropriate for patients with focal neurologic findings, seizure, or coma whose clinical features are not characteristic of TTP. In patients with clinical features consistent with TTP, imaging may not be necessary, since imaging studies typically are normal, but they may show changes consistent with reversible posterior leukoencephalopathy syndrome.
- Blood cultures: Blood cultures and other infectious disease evaluations are appropriate for those with fever or other evidence of systemic infection.
- Stool testing: Stool studies for Shiga toxin or Shiga toxin-producing organisms are indicated in individuals with severe diarrhea as the predominant clinical feature, especially bloody diarrhea.
- Tissue biopsy is not required for diagnosis, but if performed, it may show classic changes of a TMA, including platelet microthrombi in small arterioles or capillaries or hyaline changes in and around the vessel wall. Not required to distinguish TTP from other primary TMAs.

- ADAMTS13 investigation.

Screening for ADAMTS13 activity is the first test to be performed. If ADAMTS13 activity is less than 10%, TTP diagnosis is confirmed. Several assays are available for ADAMTS13 activity measurement, which in principle consists of degrading a VWF substrate, either full-length VWF (Furlan M, Robles R, Galbusera M,1998), (Tsai HM, Lian EC, 1998), (Obert B, Tout H, Veyradier A, Fressinaud E, Meyer D, Girma JP, 1999), (Gerritsen HE, Turecek PL, Schwarz HP, L¨ammle B, Furlan M, 1999) or small peptide of VWF (Kokame K, Nobe Y, Kokubo Y, Okayama A, Miyata, 2005), (Joly B, Stepanian A, Hajage D, et al. 2014) with ADAMTS13 of the tested citrated plasma or serum. Values are usually expressed as a percentage of the ADAMTS13 activity in normal pooled plasma, defined as 100%, and ideally calibrated against the new World Health Organization international standard ADAMTS13 plasma (Hubbard AR, Heath AB, Kremer Hovinga JA, 2015).

Subsequent investigations are aimed at documenting the mechanism for ADAMTS13 severe deficiency: assays for ADAMTS13 autoantibodies, searching for an ADAMTS13 inhibitor, (Furlan M, Robles R, Galbusera M,1998), (Tsai HM, Lian EC, 1998), (Veyradier A, Obert B, Houllier A, Meyer D, Girma JP, 2001) and also, in selected cases, ADAMTS13 gene sequencing. Testing for ADAMTS13 gene mutation (s) is recommended for patients with suspected hereditary TTP (Upshaw-Schulman syndrome) (e.g., positive family history, once during childhood or pregnancy, multiple recurrent episodes, absence of a demonstrable inhibitor, persistence of severe deficiency during remission).

Functional Assays for ADAMTS13

Reference methods for ADAMTS13 activity remain homemade manual methods requiring substantial skill to provide enough reliability for diagnostic use, especially because of preanalytical and analytical limitation (Ono T, Mimuro J, Madoiwa S, et al. 2006) (Gerritsen HE, Turecek PL, Schwarz HP, L¨ammle B, Furlan M., 1999). Collagen-binding activity and FRETS-VWF73-based assays are adopted reference methods for

ADAMTS13 activity measurement, (Kokame K, Nobe Y, Kokubo Y, Okayama A, Miyata T, 2005) (Knovich MA, Farland A, Owen J, 2012) whereas FRETS-VWF73 is probably superior to collagen-binding activity assay (Mancini I, Valsecchi C, Lotta LA, et al. 2014). These methods may also be time-consuming, with the shortest one (fluorescence resonance energy transfer -VWF73- assay) (Kokame K, Nobe Y, Kokubo Y, Okayama A, Miyata T, 2005) requiring several labor-intense hours for turnaround of results. As a consequence, these reference methods are limited to expert laboratories (usually 1 or 2 laboratories per country worldwide centralizing ADAMTS13 biology and networking with clinical centers involved in the management of patients with TMA). Implementation of rapid turnaround assay for ADAMTS13 activity, resulting in an accurate diagnosis with a short turnaround time, should be useful to avoid plasma exchange in patients who do not haveTTP (Connell NT, Cheves T, Sweeney JD, 2016) Inhibitory ADAMTS13 autoantibodies are also detected using functional assays (tested plasma samples are incubated with standard human plasma before residual ADAMTS13 activity measurement) (Furlan M, Robles R, Galbusera M,1998), (Tsai HM, Lian EC, 1998), (Veyradier A, Obert B, Houllier A, Meyer D, Girma JP, 2001).

Immunochemical Assays for ADAMTS13

Rapid commercial ELISA assays for ADAMTS13 activity manageable in local laboratories were recently developed, but they do not have the accuracy and the reliability of the reference methods (Thouzeau S, Capdenat S, St´epanian A, Coppo P, Veyradier, 2013) (Joly B, Stepanian A, Hajage D, et al. 2014) (Mackie I, Langley K, Chitolie A, et al. 2013) ADAMTS13 autoantibodies assays, mainly titration of anti-ADAMTS13 IgG using commercial kits (Ferrari S, Scheiflinger F, Rieger M, et al. 2007), (Moatti-Cohen M, Garrec C, Wolf M, et al. 2012) are relatively simple and are easily performed in a routine laboratory. These assays are secondary, but in the acute setting, when positive, they reinforce the diagnosis of idiopathic TTP. For all these reasons, reliable results of ADAMTS13 investigation usually cannot be available in an emergency (Sadler JE, 2015). In a large majority of cases, however, the unavailability of ADAMTS13 data in an emergency is not a limitation to initial management. Indeed, after a blood sample was quickly collected from the patient with TMA at presentation for later ADAMTS13 investigation (to avoid any interference with ADAMTS13 supplied by plasma exchange), physicians use only clinical arguments to initiate the first-line treatment in emergency. In other words, urgent therapeutic management is usually decided on the basis of TTP clinical symptoms, and not on the basis of ADAMTS13 results. (Sadler JE, 2015) (Rock GA, Shumak KH, Buskard NA, et al. 1991) (Coppo P, Froissart A, 2015) However, ADAMTS13 investigation remains crucial to definitely confirm TTP diagnosis (Sadler JE, 2015).

DIAGNOSIS

The complete "pentad" of MAHA, thrombocytopenia, fever, acute renal failure and severe neurologic findings was rare (<5%). Presence of the "pentad" was common before the routine use of therapeutic plasma exchange because the majority of patients developed progressive TMA and died from untreated disease. Therefore, the use of the "pentad" for diagnostic purposes has become obsolete.

The PTT is a clinical-hematological diagnostic entity, and there is no laboratory test that is pathognomonic.

Once MAHA and thrombocytopenia are confirmed, it is important to exclude systemic disorders as the cause of these findings. Some systemic disorders, such as severe hypertension and preeclampsia/HELLP syndrome, are obvious. However, systemic malignancies may not be initially apparent and may require other testing (ef, chest radiography, bone marrow examination) for diagnosis.

Systemic infection should be obvious, but it may mimic all clinical features of TTP and thus microbial testing may be required to identify an infectious organism.

Initiating plasma exchange (PEX) treatment for TTP is urgent. Therefore, the initial evaluation and management must balance the level of confidence in a TTP diagnosis versus the suspicion of another etiology for the MAHA and thrombocytopenia. Algorithms have been developed and validated to estimate the probability of ADMTS13 activity < 10% (and therefore the probability of the diagnosis of TTP) in a patient with MAHA and thrombocytopenia. (Bendapudi PK, Hurwitz S, Fry A, et al. 2017). Use of such an algorithm provides confidence for a diagnosis of TTP before the results of ADMTS13 activity testing is available.

A scoring system (the PLASMIC score) has been devised to predict the likelihood of ADAMTS13 activity <10% in adults (Jamme M, Rondeau E. 2017).

The clinical parameters were developed using a cohort of 214 adults with suspended thrombotic microangiopathy, and validation was performed in two additional cohorts (296 additional patients) (Jamme M, Rondeau E. 2017).

The score gives one point each for the following features:

- Platelet count <30.000/microL.
- Hemolysis (defined by reticulocyte count > 2,5%, undetectable haptoglobin, or indirect bilirubin > 2mg/dL).
- No active cancer.
- No solid organ or stem cell transplant.
- MCV <90fL.
- INR <1.5
- Creatinine < 2mg/dL.

A high PLASMIC score (6 to 7) was predictive of ADMTS13 activity of <10%, with a sensitivity of approximately 91%, this was superior to clinical judgement. A low score (0-4) suggested that ADMTS13 activity was not < 10%, with a specificity of approximately 99%. Intermediate scores (4 to 5) predict other disorders such as drug-induced thrombotic microangiopathy, disseminated intravascular coagulation, or hemolytic uremic syndrome. A score of 6 to 7 also correlated with improved survival, consistent with the diagnosis of TTP. In an independent validation of the PLASMIC score had a positive predictive value of 72%, a negative predictive value of 98%, sensitivity of 90%, and specificity of 92% (Li A,

Khalighi PR, Wu Q, Garcia DA. 2018). While this score cannot be used to definitively confirm or exclude the diagnosis of TTP, it may be helpful when there is a lack of clarity regarding the diagnosis, the role of ADMTS13 testing, an/or the need to initiate TTP therapy.

If the concern for the diagnosis of TTP is strong, then PEX may need to be initiated while the diagnostic evaluation continues. However, if the patient is not critically ill and the suspicion for the disorders discussed below is greater than the suspicion for TTP, then it may be appropriate to defer PEX while the evaluation continues. The degree of symptoms and timing of recovery with initial therapy contribute to the degree of confidence in a particular diagnosis.

A lack of early response to PEX (e.g., first three or four days) for suspended TTP encourages us to continue to seek other causes of the patient's symptoms.

SUMMARY

Primary Diagnostic Criteria

The presence of these criteria is sufficient to establish the diagnosis.

1) Microangiopathic hemolytic anemia (MAHA).
2) Thrombocytopenia.
3) Absence of cause that justifies these findings.

Other Diagnostic Criteria

These findings support the diagnosis but may be absent. All symptoms are present in 40-70% of patients1.

1) Alterations of renal function.
2) Neurological alterations.
3) Weakness
4) Abdominal symptoms.
5) Fever

CONCLUSION

1) Hereditary TTP represents <5% of all TTP cases but may be more common than acquired autoimmune TTP in certain groups such as infants or young children. Hereditary TTPA may be responsible for approximately one-fourth of episodes of TTP that occur initially during pregnancy. It is caused by homozygous or compound heterozygous mutations in the ADAMTS13 gene.
2) Acquired TTP represents 95% of all TTP cases. The median age for diagnosis is 41 years old. It is caused by the production of anti-ADAMTS13 auto-antibodies. Depending on its origin, acquired TTP may be: secondary or idiopatic.
3) Clinical features of hereditary TTP are not different from acquired TTP. Thrombocytopenia and microangiopathic hemolytic anemia characterized by schistocytes on the peripheral blood smear are consistent, defining features; neurologic abnormalities and/or renal insufficiency may also be present. Additional laboratory findings during an acute episode include increased indirect bilirubin, increased lactate dehydrogenase, and a negative direct antiglobulin (Coombs) test. Serum creatinine may be increased.
4) The patients with TTP present with a wide range of symptoms, not immediately suspicious for TTP. Unfortunately, the nonspecific nature of signs and symptoms of TTP are likely to hamper a physician's ability to suspect it on clinical grounds alone. Unless a complete blood cell count is ordered and the combination of severe thrombocytopenia and microangiopathic hemolytic anemia is noted. It is concerning that some patients may experience a delay in diagnosis.
5) ADAMTS13 is the unique specific and sensitive marker for TTP. For it correct assessment, the screening of its activity is the first test that should be performed. If ADAMTS13 activity is less than 10%, TTP diagnosis is confirmed.

6) ADAMTS13 activity ≥ 10% does not eliminate the possibility of TTP in individuals with a high confidence in the TTP diagnosis based on clinical features.
7) The unavailability of ADAMTS13 data in an emergency is not a limitation to initial management. Hence, urgent therapeutic management is usually decided on the basis of TTP clinical symptoms, and not on the basis of ADAMTS13 results. However, ADAMTS13 investigation remains crucial to definitely confirm TTP diagnosis.
8) Initiating plasma exchange (PEX) treatment for TTP is urgent, then PEX may need to be initiated while the diagnostic evaluation continues. Algorithms have been developed and validated to estimate the probability of ADMTS13 activity < 10% (and therefore the probability of the diagnosis of TTP) in a patient with MAHA and thrombocytopenia (PLASMIC score).

REFERENCES

[1] Moschcowitz E. Hyaline thrombosis of the terminal arterioles and capillaries: a hitherto undescribed disease. *Proc N Y Pathol Soc.* 1924;24:21–4.
[2] Moake JL, Rudy CK, Troll JH, Weinstein MJ, Colannino NM, Azocar J, et al. Unusually large plasma factor VIII: von Willebrand factor multimers in chronic relapsing thrombotic thrombocytopenic purpura. *N Engl J Med.* 1982;307(23):1432–5.
[3] Moake JL. Thrombotic microangiopathies. *N Engl J Med.* 2002;347(8):589–600.
[4] Furlan M, Robles R, Solenthaler M, Wassmer M, Sandoz P, Lammle B. Deficient activity of von Willebrand factor-cleaving protease in chronic relapsing thrombotic thrombocytopenic purpura. *Blood.* 1997;89:3097–103.

[5] Gerritsen HE, Robles R, Lammle B, Furlan M. Partial amino acid sequence of purified von Willebrand factor-cleaving protease. *Blood.* 2001;98(9):1654–61.

[6] Fujikawa K, Suzuki H, McMullen B, Chung D. Purification of human von Willebrand factor-cleaving protease and its identification as a new member of the metalloproteinase family. *Blood.* 2001;98(6):1662–6.

[7] Zheng X, Chung D, Takayama TK, Majerus EM, Sadler JE, Fujikawa K. Structure of von Willebrand factor-cleaving protease (ADAMTS13), a metalloprotease involved in thrombotic thrombocytopenic purpura. *J Biol Chem.* 2001;276(44):41059–63.

[8] Moatti-Cohen M, Garrec C, Wolf M, et al. Unexpected frequency of Upshaw-Schulman syndrome in pregnancy-onset thrombotic thrombocytopenic purpura. *Blood* 2012; 119:5888.

[9] Zheng XL, Kaufman RM, Goodnough LT, Sadler JE. Effect of plasma exchange on plasma ADAMTS13 metalloprotease activity, inhibitor level, and clinical outcome in patients with idiopathic and nonidiopathic thrombotic thrombocytopenic purpura. *Blood.* 2004;103(11):4043–9.

[10] Hovinga JA, Vesely SK, Terrell DR, Lammle B, George JN. Survival and relapse in patients with thrombotic thrombocytopenic purpura. *Blood.* 2010;115(8):1500–11.

[11] Vesely SK, George JN, Lämmle B, Studt JD, Alberio L, El-Harake MA, et al. ADAMTS13 activity in thrombotic thrombocytopenic purpurahemolytic uremic syndrome: relation to presenting features and clinical outcomes in a prospective cohort of 142 patients. *Blood.* 2003;102(1):60–8.

[12] Raife T, Atkinson B, Montgomery R, Vesely S, Friedman K. Severe deficiency of VWF-cleaving protease (ADAMTS13) activity defines a distinct population of thrombotic microangiopathy patients. *Transfusion.* 2004;44(2):146–50.

[13] Coppo P, Bengoufa D, Veyradier A, Wolf M, Bussel A, Millot GA, et al. Severe ADAMTS13 deficiency in adult idiopathic thrombotic microangiopathies defines a subset of patients characterized by various

autoimmune manifestations, lower platelet count, and mild renal involvement. *Medicine.* 2004;83(4):233-44.

[14] Von Krogh AS, Quist-Paulsen P, Waage A, et al. High prevalence of hereditary thrombotic thrombocytopenic purpura in central Norway: from clinical observation to evidence. *J Thromb Haemost* 2016; 14:73.

[15] Lotta LA, Garagiola I, Palla R, Cairo A, Peyvandi F. ADAMTS13 mutations and polymorphisms in congenital thrombotic thrombocytopenic purpura. *Hum Mutat.* 2010; 31: 11-9.

[16] Calderazzo JC, Kempfer A, Powazniak Y, López IR, Sánchez-Luceros A, Woods AI, Lazzari MA. A new ADAMTS13 missense mutation (D1362V) in thrombotic thrombocytopenic purpura diagnosed during pregnancy. *Thromb Haemost.* 2012; 108: 401-3.

[17] Reese JA, Muthurajah DS, Kremer Hovinga JA, et al. Children and adults with thrombotic thrombocytopenic purpura associated with severe, acquired Adamts13 deficiency: comparison of incidence, demographic and clinical features. *Pediatr Blood Cancer* 2013; 60:1676.

[18] Terrell DR, Williams LA, Vesely SK, Lämmle B, Hovinga JA, George JN. The incidence of thrombotic thrombocytopenic purpurahemolytic uremic syndrome: all patients, idiopathic patients, and patients with severe ADAMTS-13 deficiency. *J Thromb Haemost.* 2005;3(7):1432-6.

[19] Kosugi N, Tsurutani Y, Isonishi A, Hori Y, Matusmoto M, Fujimura Y. Influenza A infection triggers thrombotic thrombocytopenic purpura by producing the anti-ADAMTS13 IgG inhibitor. *Intern Med.* 2010;49:689-93.

[20] Page EE, Kremer Hovinga JA, Terrell DR, et al. Thrombotic thrombocytopenic purpura: diagnostic criteria, clinical features, and long-term outcomes from 1995 through 2015. *Blood Adv* 2017; 1:590.

[21] George JN. How I treat patients with thrombotic thrombocytopenic purpura: 2010. *Blood* 2010; 116:4060.

[22] George JN. Clinical practice. Thrombotic thrombocytopenic purpura. *N Engl J Med* 2006; 354:1927.

[23] Sadler JE, Moake JL, Miyata T, George JN. Recent advances in thrombotic thrombocytopenic purpura. *Hematology Am Soc Hematol Educ Program* 2004; 407.
[24] George JN. The importance of clinical judgment for the diagnosis of thrombotic thrombocytopenic purpura. *Transfusion* 2017; 57:2558.
[25] Scully M, Yarranton H, Liesner R, et al. Regional UK TTP registry: correlation with laboratory ADAMTS 13 analysis and clinical features. *Br J Haematol* 2008; 142:819.
[26] George JN, Nester CM. Syndromes of thrombotic microangiopathy. *N Engl J Med* 2014; 371:654.
[27] Zafrani L, Mariotte E, Darmon M, et al. Acute renal failure is prevalent in patients with thrombotic thrombocytopenic purpura associated with low plasma ADAMTS13 activity. *J Thromb Haemost* 2015; 13:380.
[28] Remuzzi G. HUS and TTP: variable expression of a single entity. *Kidney Int* 1987; 32:292.
[29] Remuzzi G. Renal involvement in patients with thrombotic thrombocytopenic purpura. *Am J Nephrol* 1986; 6:117.
[30] Hawkins BM, Abu-Fadel M, Vesely SK, George JN. Clinical cardiac involvement in thrombotic thrombocytopenic purpura: a systematic review. *Transfusion* 2008; 48:382.
[31] Gami AS, Hayman SR, Grande JP, Garovic VD. Incidence and prognosis of acute heart failure in the thrombotic microangiopathies. *Am J Med* 2005; 118:544.
[32] Patschan D, Witzke O, Dührsen U, et al. Acute myocardial infarction in thrombotic microangiopathies--clinical characteristics, risk factors and outcome. *Nephrol Dial Transplant* 2006; 21:1549.
[33] Hughes C, McEwan JR, Longair I, et al. Cardiac involvement in acute thrombotic thrombocytopenic purpura: association with troponin T and IgG antibodies to ADAMTS 13 *J Thromb Haemost* 2009; 7:529.
[34] Nokes T, George JN, Vesely SK, Awab A. Pulmonary involvement in patients with thrombotic thrombocytopenic purpura. *Eur J Haematol* 2014; 92:156.
[35] Go RS, Winters JL, Leung N, et al. Thrombotic Microangiopathy Care Pathway: A Consensus Statement for the Mayo Clinic Complement

Alternative Pathway-Thrombotic Microangiopathy (CAP-TMA) Disease-Oriented Group. *Mayo Clin Proc* 2016; 91:1189.
[36] Routh JK, Koenig SC. Severe vitamin B12 deficiency mimicking thrombotic thrombocytopenic purpura. *Blood* 2014; 124:1844.
[37] Noël N, Maigné G, Tertian G, et al. Hemolysis and schistocytosis in the emergency department: consider pseudothrombotic microangiopathy related to vitamin B12 deficiency. *QJM* 2013; 106:1017.
[38] Brain, M.C., Dacie, J.V., Hourihane, D. O'B. Microangiopathic haemolytic anaemia: the possible role of vascular lesions in pathogenesis. *Br J Haematol* 1962; 8:358.
[39] Burns ER, Lou Y, Pathak A. Morphologic diagnosis of thrombotic thrombocytopenic purpura. *Am J Hematol* 2004; 75:18.
[40] Fava S, Galizia AC. Thrombotic thrombocytopenic purpura-like syndrome in the absence of schistocytes. *Br J Haematol* 1995; 89:643.
[41] Joly, Coppo, Veyradier, *Blood,* 2017;129 (21).
[42] Furlan M, Robles R, Galbusera M, et al. von Willebrand factor-cleaving protease in thrombotic thrombocytopenic purpura and the hemolytic-uremic syndrome. *N Engl J Med.* 1998;339(22):1578-1584.
[43] Tsai HM, Lian EC. Antibodies to von Willebrand factor-cleaving protease in acute thrombotic thrombocytopenic purpura. *N Engl J Med.* 1998;339(22):1585-1594.
[44] Obert B, Tout H, Veyradier A, Fressinaud E, Meyer D, Girma JP. Estimation of the von Willebrand factor-cleaving protease in plasma using monoclonal antibodies to vWF. *Thromb Haemost.* 1999;82(5):1382-1385.
[45] Gerritsen HE, Turecek PL, Schwarz HP, L¨ammle B, Furlan M. Assay of von Willebrand factor (vWF)-cleaving protease based on decreased collagen binding affinity of degraded vWF: a tool for the diagnosis of thrombotic thrombocytopenic purpura (TTP). *Thromb Haemost.* 1999;82(5):1386-1389.
[46] Kokame K, Nobe Y, Kokubo Y, Okayama A, Miyata T. FRETS-VWF73, a first fluorogenic substrate for ADAMTS13 assay. *Br J Haematol.* 2005;129(1):93-100.

[47] Joly B, Stepanian A, Hajage D, et al. Evaluation of a chromogenic commercial assay using VWF-73 peptide for ADAMTS13 activity measurement. *Thromb Res.* 2014;134(5):1074-1080.

[48] Hubbard AR, Heath AB, Kremer Hovinga JA; Subcommittee on von Willebrand Factor. Establishment of the WHO 1st International Standard ADAMTS13, plasma (12/252): communication from the SSC of the ISTH. *J Thromb Haemost.* 2015;13(6):1151-1153.

[49] Veyradier A, Obert B, Houllier A, Meyer D, Girma JP. Specific von Willebrand factor-cleaving protease in thrombotic microangiopathies: a study of 111 cases. *Blood.* 2001;98(6):1765-1772.

[50] Ono T, Mimuro J, Madoiwa S, et al. Severe secondary deficiency of von Willebrand factor cleaving protease (ADAMTS13) in patients with sepsis-induced disseminated intravascular coagulation: its correlation with development of renal failure. *Blood.* 2006; 107(2):528-534.

[51] Kokame K, Nobe Y, Kokubo Y, Okayama A, Miyata T. FRETS-VWF73, a first fluorogenic substrate for ADAMTS13 assay. *Br J Haematol.* 2005;129(1):93-100.

[52] Knovich MA, Farland A, Owen J. Long-term management of acquired thrombotic thrombocytopenic purpura using serial plasma ADAMTS13 measurements. *Eur J Haematol.* 2012;88(6):518-525.

[53] Mancini I, Valsecchi C, Lotta LA, et al. FRETS-VWF73 rather than CBA assay reflects ADAMTS13 proteolytic activity in acquired thrombotic thrombocytopenic purpura patients. *Thromb Haemost.* 2014;112(2):297-303.

[54] Connell NT, Cheves T, Sweeney JD, 2016. Effect of ADAMTS13 activity turnaround time on plasma utilization for suspected thrombotic thrombocytopenic purpura. *Transfusion.* 2016;56(2):354-359.

[55] Thouzeau S, Capdenat S, St´epanian A, Coppo P, Veyradier A. Evaluation of a commercial assay for ADAMTS13 activity measurement. *Thromb Haemost.* 2013;110(4):852-853.

[56] Joly B, Stepanian A, Hajage D, et al. Evaluation of a chromogenic commercial assay using VWF-73 peptide for ADAMTS13 activity measurement. *Thromb Res.* 2014;134(5):1074-1080.

[57] Mackie I, Langley K, Chitolie A, et al. Discrepancies between ADAMTS13 activity assays in patients with thrombotic microangiopathies. *Thromb Haemost.* 2013;109(3):488-496.

[58] Ferrari S, Scheiflinger F, Rieger M, et al. French Clinical and Biological Network on Adult Thrombotic Microangiopathies. Prognostic value of anti-ADAMTS 13 antibody features (Ig isotype, titer, and inhibitory effect) in a cohort of 35 adult French patients undergoing a first episode of thrombotic microangiopathy with undetectable ADAMTS 13 activity. *Blood.* 2007;109(7):2815-2822.

[59] Moatti-Cohen M, Garrec C, Wolf M, et al;French Reference Center for Thrombotic Microangiopathies. Unexpected frequency of Upshaw-Schulman syndrome in pregnancy onset thrombotic thrombocytopenic purpura. *Blood.* 2012;119(24):5888-5897.

[60] Sadler JE. What's new in the diagnosis and pathophysiology of thrombotic thrombocytopenic purpura. *Hematology Am Soc Hematol Educ Program.* 2015;2015:631-636.

[61] Rock GA, Shumak KH, Buskard NA, et al; Canadian Apheresis Study Group. Comparison of plasma exchange with plasma infusion in the treatment of thrombotic thrombocytopenic purpura. *N Engl J Med.* 1991;325(6):393-397.

[62] Coppo P, Froissart A, French Reference Center for Thrombotic Microangiopathies. Treatment of thrombotic thrombocytopenic purpura beyond therapeutic plasma exchange. *Hematology Am Soc Hematol Educ Program.* 2015;2015:637-643.

[63] Bendapudi PK, Hurwitz S, Fry A, et al. Derivation and external validation of the PLASMIC score for rapid assessment of adults with thrombotic microangiopathies: a cohort study. *Lancet Haematol* 2017; 4:e157.

[64] Jamme M, Rondeau E. The PLASMIC score for thrombotic thrombocytopenic purpura. *Lancet Haematol* 2017; 4:e148.

[65] Li A, Khalighi PR, Wu Q, Garcia DA. External validation of the PLASMIC score: a clinical prediction tool for thrombotic thrombocytopenic purpura diagnosis and treatment. *J Thromb Haemost* 2018; 16:164.

Chapter 3

DIFFERENTIAL DIAGNOSIS AND TREATMENT OF THROMBOTIC THROMBOCYTOPENIC PURPURA

Martin Antonio Cabero - Becerra[1,], MD,*
Lorena Picó Rico[1], MD,
Ana Dolores Del Rey Lujan[1], MD,
Carmen Cristina Amorós Pérez[2], MD
and Llanos Belmonte Andújar[3], MD

[1]Hematology and Hemotherapy,
Hospital of Alcázar de San Juan, Ciudad Real, Spain
[2]Hematology and Hemotherapy, Hospital Virgen de los Lirios,
Alcoy, Alicante, Spain
[3]Obstetrics and Gynecology Department,
Hospital of Almansa, Albacete, Spain

---

[*] Corresponding Author's E-mail: marcabero@hotmail.com.

Abstract

Thrombotic thrombocytopenic purpura (TTP) is usually diagnosed with thrombocytopenia, microangiopathic hemolytic anemia, neuropathy, renal failure, and fever, although thrombocytopenia, schistocytes in the peripheral blood smear, and high levels of Lactic dehydrogenase (LDH) are sufficient for diagnosis. ADAMTS13 serum levels are very low and the coagulation study is usually normal, in contrast to other diseases.

Thrombocytopenia of TTP is usually moderate, secondary to thrombotic microangiopathies (TMA). In addition, other pathologies may have moderate thrombocytopenia and must be differentiated. Indeed, the most frequent are hemolytic uremic syndrome associated with infection (HUS), HELLP syndrome and disseminated intravascular coagulation (DIC). There are other pathologies with moderate thrombocytopenia that we should consider, such as hereditary TTP, hereditary SHU, TMA associated with some medications, transplantation or hidden malignancies. The accuracy of the diagnosis is fundamental to be able to give the most effective treatment possible, to improve the long-term results.

The usual treatment of autoimmune TTP is plasma exchange, using fresh frozen or cryoprecipitated plasma, eliminating vWF multimers of high molecular weight and providing ADAMTS13. In some cases, rituximab is effective in this condition, and we can use it together with the plasma exchange, which reduces the risk of relapse. In refractory cases, or in which relapse is frequent, high doses of corticosteroids, vincristine, intravenous immunoglobulin or immunosuppressive therapy, such as azathioprine or cyclophosphamide, would be used.

In cases of HUS, renal support dialysis and control of hypertension are the pillars of the treatment. Platelet transfusions are contraindicated in HUS and TTP. For the atypical SUH, the treatment is similar to renal insufficiency, but we can add Eculizumab to inhibit the activation of the complement.

Mortality is approximately 90% in non-treated cases for that reason a Clinical suspicion and a correct diagnosis is essential. The objective of this chapter is to indicate the most reliable tests collected from the literature, with the purpose of an early and accurate diagnosis, which is fundamental to administer the most appropriate treatment.

Introduction

Thrombotic microangiopathies (TMAs), specially, thrombotic thrombocytopenic purpura (TTP) and hemolytic uremic syndrome (HUS) are acute life-threatening disorders that require prompt consideration, diagnosis, and treatment to improve the high morbidity and mortality. Differentiating TTP from other TMAs can be difficult given their significant overlap in clinical presentations.

If a patient presents with thrombocytopenia and anemia in the laboratory, TTP or and another TMA should be ruled out. Specifically, in this case, we have to review a blood film and undertaking hemolytic parameters. We can see schistocytes and, often, polychromasia in the peripheral blood smear. Confirmation of an underlying hemolytic process includes an increase in lactate dehydrogenase (LDH), reticulocytosis, and low or absent haptoglobin. In contrast to other hemolytic anemias, the direct antiglobulin test must be negative in TTP.

Clinically, the presentation is with microangiopathic hemolytic anemia and thrombocytopenia (MAHAT) and variable organ symptoms resulting from microvascular thrombi. Patients may present neurological symptoms (such as stroke, transient ischemic attacks, migraines, and seizures), renal impairment, abdominal pain, and cardiac involvement. A diagnosis of TTP is confirmed by a sever deficiency in ADAMT13 (a disinterring and metalloproteinase with a thrombospondin type 1 motif, member 13). The determination of ADAMTS13 may be delayed in time according to the hospital where the patient is admitted. However, without treatment, the mortality in TTP is 90% (Scully, 2017). Therefore, the plasma exchange (PEX) should be initiated as soon as possible after consideration or these TMA.

Nevertheless, there are other medical situations that are presented as MAHAT and should be excluded to start the specific treatment of the disease as soon as possible, since this has a critical impact on outcome (Scully & Goodship, 2014). Next, we will disregard the main medical conditions to be taken into account in the diagnosis of TTP (Table 1), and its treatment.

Table 1. Differential diagnosis of TTP form others TMAs

Condition	Comments
TTP Congenital TTP Acquired TTP	Mutations in ADAMTS13. Typically in pregnancy (infection/neonatal period may be associated with younger diagnoses) Presence of antibodies to ADAMS13
HUS Complement mediated Infection-associated	Exclude STEC and non-STEC. HUS presenting up to 7 days following hemorrhagic colitis. Confirm by serology/PCR, also pneumococcus, HIV and viral associated. Genetic analysis may confirm complement mutations. Shigatoxin-producing E. Coli (STEC), shigella, pneumococci, etc.
DIC	Thrombocytopenia is often the initial feature. Coagulation abnormalities are variable, but associated low fibrinogen suggests severity. Sepsis, malignancy, trauma, hematological disorders, obstetric complications.
Malignancy-associated TMA	TMA maybe de initial feature of a cancer presentation or in relation to drugs required to treat active cancer. Usually disseminated breast, lung and gastric cancers, or hematological malignancies.
DA-TMA	A number of drugs very rarely associated with antibody-mediated TTP (Table 2). Gemcitabine, mitomycin and anti-VEGF therapy may associated with an HUS-type picture.
TA-TMA	Solid organs and hematopoietic stem cell transplantation, results from endothelial cell damage, from underlying conditioning therapies, immunosuppressive, or complications relating to the transplant (e.g., graft-versus-host disease).
Infections	May precipitate TTP or HUS. Viral, bacterial, or fungal infections associated to endothelia cells damage. Confirmation by serology, culture or PCR. Treat underlying infection.
Malignant hypertension	Primary or in association with a specific disorder (e.g., IgA nephropathy). Cannot reliably differentiate form CH-HUS, especially if normal renal size or radiological examination and no chronic features of high blood pressure.
Pregnancy associated	HELLPS or PET. Deliver baby usually helps to resolution, but if progressive symptoms/worsening laboratory parameters, considers TTP or HUS.
Autoimmune disease/vasculitis	Relevant immunology investigations +/- biopsy will confirm. Normal ADAMTS13 levels.
B12 deficiency	Anemia, reticulocytosis, thrombocytopenia, but typical MAHA features not present. Vitamin B12 deficiency. Care review of blood film.

DIFFERENTIAL DIAGNOSIS

Hemolytic Uremic Syndrome (HUS)

TTP and HUS exist on a spectrum. HUS is best described under the practical and inclusive term of TMA. Although HUS shares the definition of a MAHA with thrombocytopenia and microvascular thrombosis, HUS additionally includes prominent renal impairment or failure (Noris y Remuzzi 2005).

To complicate the concept of TMAs further is the emergence of typical and atypical HUS definitions. Typical HUS is also called infection-associated HUS (iaHUS) and is characterized by HUS syndrome with bloody diarrhea, and it is associated with Shiga toxin-producing Escherichia Coli (STEC), typically serotype O157:H7. This source was implicated in 73% to 83% of HUS cases in major epidemiologic studies (Banatvala, et al. 2001). But also, other non-0157 serotypes, as well as Shiga toxin-secreting strains, including *Shigella* and *Campylobacter* (Tarr, Gordon and Chandler 2005). It results from ingestion of infected water of food or person to person. The median incubation period is 3 to 4 days. Cases may present with bloody diarrhea, but the TMA usually presents 4 to 7 days after this has resolved. The toxin acts on vascular endothelium, specifically binding to glycolipid globotriaosylceramide (Gb3) receptors, particularly in the glomerulus of the kidney and, therefore, associated with acute kidney injury. Children are more commonly affected with a mortality of 5% to 10% (Majowicz, et al. 2014). A small percentage of cases of HUS are caused by *Streptococcus pneumoniae*, which are more likely to be associated with pneumonia and may lead to multiorgan failure.

Atypical HUS (aHUS) is characterized by laboratory characteristics similar to those of HUS and may have diarrhea, but not necessarily bloody, and its underlying pathophysiology is due to the activation and regulation of the deficient complement system, therefore, the atypical HUS is also known as complement-mediated HUS (CM-HUS) (Tsai 2013). aHUS resulting from a gain-of-function mutation of complement C3 of factor B or a loss-of-function mutation of complement factor H, factor I, membrane cofactor protein or thrombomodulin (Fremeaux-Bacchi, et al. 2013) or by platelet activation as a results of the mutations in diacylglycerol kinase epsilon (DGKE) (Lemaire, et al. 2013). However, only about 50% of aHUS cases have identifiable genetic abnormalities and 1-2% of aHUS patients may have autoantibodies against to complement factor H (CFH). The underlying etiologies for the other 50% of aHUS cases are yet to be identified (Marina y Remuzzi 2009). Clinically, an infectious precipitant may need excluding. A viral or bacterial trigger or vaccination may be associated with presentation.

Typical HUS is treated with supportive care, which includes blood transfusions when needed, judicious control of hypertension (preferably with nifedipine or nicardipine), careful maintenance of fluids and electrolytes, and hemodialysis when clinically indicated (Tarr, Gordon and Chandler 2005). Dialysis was required in 63% of patients with HUS in one study (Gerber, et al. 2002). In a meta-analysis of treatment modalities for typical HUS, there was no difference in mortality or clinical outcome when supportive care was compared with FFP infusion, anticoagulation medications, steroids, or a Shiga-toxin-binding agent (Michael, et al. 2009). PEX therapy lacks compelling support in children with typical HUS and is controversial in adults (Menne, et al. 2012), but it may be considered when severe neurologic abnormalities are present.

Atypical HUS is often hard to distinguish from TTP in the acute care setting and should be treated as a closed TTP variant with PEX therapy until a definitive diagnosis can be determined. In atypical HUS, Eculizumab, an inhibitor to complement C5, is increasing used (Mannuci 2013).

Mortality has been up to 25% with high rates of end-stage renal failure within 1 year (Nester, et al. 2015).

DISSEMINATED INTRAVASCULAR COAGULATION (DIC)

Disseminated intravascular coagulation (DIC) is the secondary disorder that most often presents as a TMA (Barcellini, et al. 2014). DIC is a serious disease that causes microvascular thrombosis associated with thrombocytopenia, a tendency to bleeding and organ failure. These symptoms and laboratory data are similar to those of the microangiopathic thrombotic and we should be able to distinguish it from TTP (Wada, et al. 2018). According to the International Society of Thrombosis and Haemostasis (ISTH), DIC is an acquired syndrome characterized by the intravascular activation of coagulation and consumption of the coagulation. It is an acquired, systemic process of overstimulation of the coagulation pathway resulting in thrombosis, followed by consumption of platelets and coagulation factors, and ending in hemorrhage. DIC is characterized by the generation of fibrin related markers (soluble fibrin monomers, fibrinogen and fibrin degradation products, D-dimers, etc.) and reflects an acquired (inflammatory) or non- inflammatory disorder of the microvasculature. DIC can be acute and decompensated when the generation of clotting factor cannot match the excessive consumption, or chronic and compensated when the clotting factor consumption is matched by production (Fletcher B, et al. 2001).

Patients with DIC may show characteristics of TMA with the underlying bases, which include severe trauma, sepsis, malignancy, preeclampsia/HELLP syndrome, etc. Therefore, DIC is often associated with TMA and TMA is often associated with DIC (Schwameis, et al. 2015). There may be acute renal failure; jaundice, thromboembolism, coma, delirium, headache, neurological deficits and shock can be present. DIC is a clinical diagnosis, but the laboratory data can help in the presumptive diagnosis (Kappler, et al. 2014). Because of the consumptive coagulopathy, patients with DIC have prolonged prothrombin time and activated partial thromboplastin time, elevated fibrin degradation products or D-dimer, reduced fibrinogen, and increase thrombin time. Thrombocytopenia, which is often the first and most sensitive sing of DIC, is present in >90% of cases with 50% of cases having a platelet count >50 x 10^9/L. A reduced platelet count is associated with increased thrombin formation and amplified fibrinolytic activity, associated with raised D-dimers. There is variability in derangement of the coagulation test in 60% to 70% of case, but the may be normal o indeed shortened. Fibrinogen may be reduced, but it is less commonly below the normal laboratory range unless there is very sever DIC.

The sequential changes in these parameters may be more helpful in confirming a diagnosis of DIC. Markedly decreased ADAMSTS13 levels have been reported in severe sepsis patients without TTP, suggesting that platelet activation due to decreased ADAMST13 might be observed in DIC patients with severe sepsis (Wada, et al. 2018).

Unlike TTP, there is no gold standard for diagnosing DIC or a specific biomarker that clearly diagnoses DIC, so they can be diagnosed using a scoring system that uses global coalition tests. Various scoring systems are available for diagnosis of DIC, including one developed by the ISTH (Levi, et al. 2009).

This scoring system should only be used in patients with an underlying disorder that is known to cause DIC; prospective studies in an intensive care unit setting showed that the ISTH scoring system had a sensitivity of 91% and a specificity of 97% for de diagnosis of DIC. Thus, in appropriate clinical situations, DIC should be ruled out, given that a significantly low ADAMTS13 activity (<10 IU dL^{-1}) may occur (Saha, McDaniel and Zheng 2017).

The prognosis for those with DIC is poor and up to 50% of patients will die. DIC from sepsis has a significantly higher death rate than DIC associated with trauma (Kappler, et al. 2014). The only effective treatment for DIC is the reversal of the underlying cause.

In patients with sepsis, there is no scientific evidence that platelet prophylactic transfusion is effective in the prevention of bleeding or in the reduction of mortality (Lieberman L, et al. 2014). The cause of thrombocytopenia in these patients is usually multifactorial, associating a higher peripheral consumption and a reduced marrow production. Although thrombopenic patients seem to have a higher mortality, platelet transfusion should be reserved for prophylaxis only in case of invasive techniques, and as a treatment for patients with moderate hemorrhage (Jimenez-Marco, et al. 2015).

Platelet therapeutic transfusion will be made when there is a quantitative and/or qualitative alteration of the platelets and active bleeding attributable to the platelet defect. In patients with DIC the attitude towards the presence of hemorrhage and thrombocytopenia, apart from treating the cause of it will be to maintain a figure >50 x 10^9/L platelets (Jimenez-Marco, et al. 2015).

Heparin augments antithrombin III activity and prevents conversion of fibrinogen to fibrin. Heparin should only be used when there is evidence of thromboembolic disease, retained products of conception or purpura fulminant (gangrene of digits and extremities) and requires a normal antithrombin level be preinitiation. Fresh Frozen Plasma (FFP) contains coagulation factors as well as Protein C and Protein S and is recommended with significant, active bleeding and a fibrinogen level less than 100mg/dL. The administration of antithrombin III concentrate has a theoretical benefit, but currently there is no validated mortality benefit (Levi, de Jonge and van der Poll 2004).

MALIGNANCY-ASSOCIATED TMA

TMA may be the presenting feature of an underlying cancer, either in undiagnosed disease or in association with metastases. The estimated incidence is between 0.25 and 0.45 cases per million residents (Lechner K, 2012), lower than that of autoimmune TTP. TMA can occur to multiple causes: obstruction of the microcirculation through the invasion of cancer cells, microvascular thrombosis, DIC and chemotherapeutic agents. In one of the largest reviews of cancer-associated microangiopathy, more than 90% of the cases showed metastatic cancer when TMA was diagnosed; 24% of patients had neurological or renal involvement, 36% had leucoerythroblastic presentation on peripheral smear, and 36% had low fibrinogen with elevated fibrin degradations products or D-dimer, suggestive of DIC (Lechner K, 2012).

Majority of cases are solid tumor malignancies, but hematological cancers such as lymphoma make up approximately 8% of all cases. The most likely diagnosis is gastric, lung, breast and prostate, mainly adenocarcinoma. Respiratory symptoms were more commonly presented (unlike TTP or HUS) (Barcellini W, 2014).

The activity of ADAMTS13 plasma in the TMA associated with malignancy is usually normal or moderately reduced (35-84 UL dL^{-1}) (Fontana S, 2001). In some cases with IgG antibody was reported severe deficiency of ADAMSTS13 activity (<10 IU dL^{-1}) (J. George 2011).

Distinguishing cancer-associated TMA form TTP may be difficult initially, but the former is likelier to have respiratory symptoms and bone pain at presentation. Therefore, the presence of TMA with any of the following clinical characteristics, including advanced age, history of cancer, pulmonary involvement (e.g., pleural effusion and interstitial infiltration), extreme elevation of serum LDH, laboratory analytical characteristics of CID and symptoms of progressive constitutional syndrome, should provoke an exhaustive search for a hidden malignancy (J. George 2011). Review of the peripheral blood smear and a bone marrow aspirate may help expedite the underlying cancer diagnosis.

Treatment with antitumor therapy was associated with improved survival, and there was no role for plasma therapy, steroids or other immunosuppressive used in TTP (Lechner K, 2012); but the use of platelet transfusions for severe thrombocytopenia, generally contraindicated in TTP, would be appropriate.

DRUG-ASSOCIATED TMA (DA-TMA)

The use of some drugs (Table 2) has been described as a cause of TMA (Al-Nouri, et al. 2015). The most definitive cause of DA-TMA was with ticlopidine (Kupfer and Tessler 1997). Ticlopidine is an antiplatelet agent derived from thienopyridine, as is clopidogrel. The TMA associated with ticlopidine occurs in the first weeks after the start of treatment. These patients usually present a severe deficiency of ADAMTS13 activity as a consequence of the appearance of autoantibodies against ADAMTS13. Therefore, they respond to plasma exchange therapy (Bennett, et al. 2013). TMA associated with clopidogrel also occurs in the first weeks but does not seem to be associated with a severe ADAMTS13 deficiency or with detectable inhibitors, therefore, plasma exchange will generally not be effective (Jacob S, et al. 2012). Similarly, quinine can cause immune-mediated TMA with acute kidney injury and may also cause liver toxicity or DIC. In this case, patients should improve with plasma exchange and prednisone (Gottschall, et al. 1991).

The pathophysiology of DA-TMAs is varied. In some cases, mechanisms include antibodies, for example, to red cells or platelets, such as with oxaliplatin (Phan, et al. 2009). Drugs targeting specific proteins, such as vascular endothelial growth factor (VEGF) inhibitors, cause hypertension and microthrombi formation exclusive to glomerular capillaries (Grangé and Coppo 2017). TMA secondary to anti-VEGF therapy tends to present as hypertension, proteinuria and, rarely, renal failure. ADAMTS13 is usually normal or slightly low (>20 IU dL^{-1}) in such cases (Izzedine H, et al. 2014).

Some TMAs occur as a result of cumulative toxicity, such as with mitomycin and gemcitabine. The mechanism is unclear and can be due to a direct effect on endothelial cells and tend to cause kidney damage and uncontrolled blood pressure (Medina, Sipols and George 2001).

Table 2. Drugs associated with thrombotic microangiopathy

Ticlodopine
Estrogen-containing durgs
Quinine
Gemcitabine
Mitomycin C
VEGF inhititors (e.g., bevacizumab, aflibercept)
Proteosome inhibitors (e.g., carfilzomib and bortezomib)
Thyrosine kinase inhibitors
Interferon-β
Calcineurin inhibitors (e.g., ciclosporin, tacrolimus)
Platinum-based drugs (e.g., oxaliplatin)
Emicizumab (in conjunt with bypassing agents)

Cyclosporine and tacrolimus, calcineurin inhibitors (CNIs) such as used as immunosuppressive drugs after solid or hematology transplantation, can also cause TMA that more resembles aHUS.

The main treatment for DA-TMA is the suspension of the offensive drug. PEX is often done but of uncertain utility, as only a small proportion are associated with antibodies to ADAMTS13 (Anaadriana Zakarija, 2012). There have been case reports/smalls series demonstrating a possible beneficial effect of rituximab and eculizumab in refractory cases of chemotherapy induces TMA (Izzedine, et al. 2006).

TRANSPLANT-ASSOCIATED TMA (TA-TMA)

Patients with solid organ or hematopoietic stem cell transplant (HSCT) may present with TMAs. The underlying pathology is endothelial damage (Jodele, et al. 2015), which can be caused by previous conditioning therapies, HLA- mismatched transplant, graft-versus-host disease, humoral rejection and medication. Medications, including CNIs, antiVEGF bevacizumab and sirolimus, have been implicated in TMA in this patiens (George, et al. 2012). TMA associated with transplantations most commonly affects the kidneys but can manifest with gastrointestinal, pulmonary, neurological or cardiac involvement. Antybody-mediated rejection in a renal allograft can have similar histological features to TMA. Predomiant endarteritis, presence of C4d staining of peritubular capilaries, and donor-specific (Noris y Remuzzi 2010). Typically has normal or midly low ADAMTS13 activity. Recently, inhcrited or acquired defect in complement have been identified and thougt to compound the endothelial damage.

It is important to consider an additional uderlyin infection such as adenovirus, indeed, nearly 50% of patients at post mortem relating to HSCT had evidence of viremia, with some cases only diagnosed at post mortem (Kojouri & George, 2008).

Some parameters as asocieated with encreased mortality like proteinuria, raised LDH and hypertension (Jodele, Davies, et al. 2014). It is not benefit of PEX and treatment is bases on symptomatic support. The use of complement inhibitor therapy has been associated with positive results in some case small series (Cavero, et al. 2007) (Rosenthal 2016).

INFECTIONS-ASSOCIATED TMA

Systemic bacterial, viral or fungal infections can cause MAHA and thrombocytopenia and therefore should always be considered during evaluation of such patients. On the other hand, an infection can also trigger an acute episode of TTP, as has been observed with the influenza virus (Jonsson, et al. 2015), and it can be difficult to differentiate whether the infection is the cause or a trigger

ADAMTS13 activity in patients with TMA associated with infection is usually normal (>20 IU dL^{-1}), although severe deficiency of ADAMTS13 has also been observed in the absence of an inhibitor in severe sepsis, dengue, endocarditis and sepsis-induced DIC (Ono, et al. 2006). The underlying mechanism is multifactorial but is thought to be due to endothelial damage leading to increased VWF release and increased consumption of ADAMTS13, bacterial enzymes leading to ADAMTS13 proteolysis, and cytokine-mediated protease inhibition (Schwameis, et al. 2015). In addition, extracellular neutrophil traps (NETs), chromatin fibers (containing histones and antimicrobial proteins) released from neutrophils during infection or inflammation can result in thrombosis due to their ability to aggregate and platelet adhesion. Elevated NETs markers have been demonstrated in the patient's plasma during the acute episode of TMA (Fuchs, et al. 2012).

HIV may present with TTP, severe ADAMTS13 deficiency, and an immune-mediated pathogenesis. Advanced disease with opportunistic infections (HHV-8 and CMV), malignant neoplasms (Kaposi's sarcoma) and antiviral drugs can trigger a TMA. In addition, during immune reconstitution with initiation of highly active antiretroviral therapy, elevated levels of cytokines (IL-6 and IL-8) may inhibit ADAMTS-13 activity and result in features of TMA (George, et al. 2012). Plasma apheresis should be considered in an HIV patient who has features of TMA in the presence of severe ADAMTS13 deficiency provided other opportunistic infections, malignancies and other causes have been ruled out.

Many other infections can present with a TMA, but require a careful assessment of the history, microbiology and virology.

MALIGNANT HYPERTENSION ASSOCIATED TMA

Malignant hypertension may mimic presentation of CM-HUS. Severely elevated blood pressure with associated retinal changes (i.e., papilledema, flame-shape hemorrhage, cotton wool spots) is a characteristic feature of malignant hypertension. Patients with malignant hypertension may present with MAHA, thrombocytopenia and renal failure; conversely, patients with TMA sometimes can also present with severe hypertension, especially those with renal involvement. Patients with malignant hypertension presented with a mean systolic blood pressure of 160 mmHg, renal failure and schistocytes in blood smear and a modest reduction of platelet count (mean 60×10^9/L). Plasma ADAMTS13 activity usually >10 IU dL^{-1}. The reduced ADAMTS-13 activity might be caused by consumption related to endothelial activation and increased levels of plasma VWF (Khanal, et al. 2015). The TMA associated with hypertension improves after aggressive control of blood pressure and controlling blood pressure should be the main objective in these cases.

PREGNANCY-ASSOCIATED TMA

Pregnancy-associated TMAs includes specific conditions, e.g., TTP or HUS precipitated by pregnancy, or TMAs particular to pregnancy, such as pre-eclampsia, hemolysis, elevated liver enzymes, and low platelets, or acute fatty liver (AFL) of pregnancy. The incidence of pregnancy-associated TMAs may be greater than originally anticipated. Indeed, 5% of all causes of pregnant women with a platelet count <75×10^9/L during pregnancy have been identified as congenital TTP (Delmas, et al. 2015). The level of VWF increase during pregnancy with a concomitant decrease in ADAMTS13 activity, mainly due to consumption or related to estrogen, in the second and third trimester that persists for a few weeks postpartum (Scully, Hunt, et al. 2012). Some situations associated with pregnancy can precipitate TMA, such as ovarian stimulation, viral infection, thyroiditis, HIV, lupus or antiphospholipid syndrome (APS) (Moatti-Cohen, et al. 2012).

Differentiating TTP or aHUS during pregnancy may be difficult as both conditions can be associated with hypertension, proteinuria, and intrauterine growth retardation. The possibility of TTP and aHUS should be considered in patients with thrombocytopenia, particularly with a platelet count <50 x 10^9/L. Determination elevation LDH can be a help in this distinction, since this is not altered by normal pregnancy.

Both TTP and aHUS can occur during pregnancy and after delivery. TTP can present at any stage during pregnancy or in the postpartum period, but most commonly, it does so in the third trimester, whereas acute fatty liver (AFL) and HELLP syndrome typically occur in the second and third trimesters. The presence of sever renal injury may be more suggestive of aHUS or HELLP syndrome than TTP, and in thought to be most common in the postpartum period. Acute renal injury in HELLP syndrome is usually associated with acute tubular necrosis without thrombosis, which may improve with conservative management (Fakhouri 2016). Symptoms of headache, fever, abdominal pain and nausea may be seen in many different TMAs, but hypoglycemia is no a presenting feature of TTP or aHUS and may be more suggestive of AFL or HELLP syndrome.

It is important to determine the level of ADAMTS13 on the first day of presentation before the start of plasma therapy. An ADAMTS13 activity <10 IU dL^{-1} with or without autoantibody is a diagnosis for TTP. Plasma infusion therapy or exchange therapy should be initiated immediately upon suspicion of TTP.

AUTOIMMUNE DISEASE/VASCULITIS

A variety of autoimmune/vasculitis conditions may present as a trigger to TTP or may have MAHAT features. Conectivopathies can present with a TMA. For example, acute scleroderma is differentiated by clinical features and may present with or without severe renal involvement, simulating TTP or HUS (Woodworth, et al. 2016).

Other diseases that can simulate TTP are systemic lupus erythematosus (SLE), antiphospholipid syndrome or vasculitis, such as lupus nephritis or Goodpasture syndrome. To exclude an underlying connective tissue disease, confirmation by relevant autoantibodies is required, but should be cautious with this, since there are a number of patients with TMA who have a positive autoantibody test, especially antinuclear antibodies, who do not have SLE. Biopsy tissue can help to confirm the diagnoses, and ADAMTS13 levels will be normal in this case. Underlying autoimmune diseases should be excluded for TTP and HUS presentations (Roriz, et al. 2015).

Others

A cause of TMA to be attention is vitamin B12 deficiency, that is an uncommon but eminently treatable disorder. The laboratory parameters at presentation may be identical to TTP, with anemia, raised reticulocytes and thrombocytopneia, but the blood film finding are not specifically in keeping with MAHA. Patients respond quickly to B12 injections. Further follow-up to exclude pernicious anemia with intrinsic factor antibodies or celiac disease. Therefore, it is proposed that B12 and folate levels are assumed as part is routine screening for acute TMAs (Scully 2017).

TREATMENT OF ACQUIRED THROMBOTIC THROMBOCYTOPENIC PURPURA

Therapy should be initiated if the diagnosis of aTTP is seriously considered (Paul Coppo and Veyradier 2012), because is a medical emergency that is almost always fatal if appropriate treatment is not initiated promptly; with appropriate treatment, survival rates of up to 90 percent are possible (Bell et al. 1991).

Plasma Exchange (PEX)

PEX works by replacing ADAMTS13 and removing the autoantibodies that are inhibiting ADAMTS13 activity as well as any residual ultra large VWF multimers. Correcting ADAMTS13 deficiency in turn restores proper cleavage of ultra large von Willebrand factor (vWF) multimers, prevents microvascular thrombosis, and reverses symptoms of organ damage (Moake 2002) (Byrnes et al. 1990).

ADAMTS13 measurement to guide the use of plasma exchange in patients with TTP is controversial. In one study, plasma exchange was initiated only in patients with ADAMTS13 activity < 10%. Not initiating PEX in patients without severe ADAMTS13 deficiency proved to be a safe approach, with no increase in mortality (Shah et al. 2013).

As we know the establishment of the treatment as soon as possible is crucial, because aTTP is a medical emergency, the prolonged waiting for the results of the test, in practice, prevent its use in the decision to start the plasma exchange, which does not it means that if this test is available, it should also be requested.

We have available for the realization of PEX, Fresh frozen plasma (FFP), Thawed plasma, Cryoprecipitate reduced plasma and pathogen-inactivated products such as solvent-treated/detergent-treated plasma (S/D) or treated with amotosalen-UVA. Some clinicians prefer to use specific products; as an example, in the United Kingdom and Canada, S/D Plasma is used almost exclusively due to the potential for reduced viral transmission (Blombery and Scully 2014).

The start of treatment depends on the clinician, the protocol used in the reference health center and the experience in the management of aTTP. The mainstay of treatment for aTTP is daily plasma exchange therapy (PEX) with fresh frozen plasma, preferably within 4 – 8 hours, according to British TTP guidelines (Scully et al. 2012) and the Canadian apheresis trial (Rock et al. 1991). Although PEX remains the treatment of choice, large volume plasma infusions are indicated if there is to be a delay in arranging PEX (Duffy and Coyle 2013).

The duration of PEX and the number of procedures required to achieve remission is highly variable but is longer in antibody-mediated TTP (Coppo et al. 2006). An optimal regimen has not been determined. In the Canadian apheresis trial, 1 – 5 x Plasma Volume (PV) exchange was performed on the first 3 days followed by 1 – 0 PV exchange thereafter (Rock et al. 1991).

More intensive exchange, such as twice daily PEX, may be required in resistant cases especially if there is new symptomatology, such as neurological or cardiac events. Daily exchanges should continue for a minimum of 2 days after complete remission, defined as normal platelet count (>150 x 10^9/l). Tapering (reducing frequency and/or volume of PEX) has not been shown to reduce relapse rates (Bandarenko et al. 1998).

Corticosteroids

As the trigger is an immunological disorder, many centers initiate high doses of corticosteroids at the same time as plasma exchange. Higher dose pulsed steroids have shown to be associated with an improved patient outcome and usually have minimal side effects (Balduini et al. 2010). British TTP guidelines, recommended Intravenous daily methyl-prednisolone (e.g., 1 g/d for three consecutive days – adult dose) or high dose oral prednisolone (e.g., 1 mg/kg/d) should be considered (Scully et al. 2012).

Rituximab

Rituximab is a chimeric monoclonal antibody directed against CD20, a cell surface protein in mature B cells that was initially used for the treatment of non-Hodgkin's lymphoma. Currently, it is also used as an immunosuppressive agent in several autoimmune disorders, including aTTP, but it is used off label.

It is an effective curative therapy in patients with acute refractory aTTP related to anti-ADAMTS13 antibodies and a promising prophylactic treatment in selected patients with severe relapsing aTTP and persistent anti-ADAMTS13 antibodies (Fakhouri et al. 2005), and was associated with a prompt remission, despite their failure to respond to PEX and methylprednisolone alone (Scully et al. 2007).

The optimal dose of rituximab has not been established in aTTP, therefore the dose of lymphoproliferative disorders is used, although there is currently evidence to support the low dose of rituximab because in other autoimmune cytopenias it seems to be effective.

Typically, 375 mg/m2 has been used weekly for 4 weeks. Patients receiving rituximab showed reductions in anti-ADAMTS13 IgG antibody levels and increased ADAMTS13 activity (Scully et al. 2007). One study, showed than upfront low dose rituximab for aTTP were associated with low rates of early exacerbation or refractory aTTP, favorable outcomes compared with historical controls, incidence of refractory or exacerbations was 12% at 30 days, relapse rate of 28% at 2 years, and adverse events were observed with low dose rituximab (Westwood et al. 2017). Other study, showed than the risk of relapse appears to be reduced with rituximab use (Heidel et al. 2007).

Ideally PEX should be withheld for at least 4 hours after completing a rituximab infusion (Scully et al. 2007). Giving rituximab more frequently than weekly e.g., every 3–4 d, may overcome removal during PEX (McDonald et al. 2010). There is no evidence of increased infection risk with rituximab in aTTP patients.

Rituximab has been routinely administered as a second-line treatment, when patients became refractory or relapsed, and it was recommended in acute idiopathic TTP with neurological/cardiac pathology, which are associated with a high mortality, rituximab should be considered on admission, in conjunction with PEX and steroids (Scully et al. 2012).

Predictors of relapse and efficacy of rituximab in aTTP remain unclear. Use of Rituximab was associated with short-term protection from relapse but not long-term relapse free survival. Age, non-O blood group, and prior aTTP were significantly associated with an increased risk of relapse (Sun et al. 2018).

Currently, has shown benefit in using rituximab as a first line therapy at presentation of aTTP (Scully et al. 2011) and there are evidence to support relapse pre-emptive therapy (Hie et al. 2014). It reduced relapse rates when used as initial therapy for TTP (Page et al. 2016), appeared to be associated with faster attainment of remission and fewer PEX treatments than later rituximab (Lim, Vesely, and George 2015).

Splenectomy

It is used in refractory cases and relapsing aTTP but has limited proven benefit (Scully et al. 2012).

Antiplatelet Agents

The clinical efficacy of antiplatelet agents in aTTP is unproven but they are relatively safe. Low dose aspirin (75 mg OD) may be given during platelet recovery (platelet count >50 x 10^9/l) (Scully et al. 2012).

N-Acetylcysteine

N-acetylcysteine (NAC) was recently suggested as a potential therapeutic adjunct for patients with aTTP. Utilization of NAC in the management of aTTP either as an adjunctive treatment in cases refractory to PEX or part of the initial treatment regimen including PEX and steroids, in patients with severe presentation. Based upon their severe presentation or lack of response to initial treatment with PEX, corticosteroids and other immunosuppressive agents, NAC was added. In a case reports under this combined treatment, all patients had a significant clinical improvement of symptoms with concurrent normalization of platelet count and ADAMTS13 activity level. This report highlights the potential therapeutic utility of NAC in the treatment of aTTP (Rottenstreich et al. 2016).

Bortezomib

It has been a breakthrough in the treatment of multiple myeloma, proteasome inhibition could also be effective in the management of aTTP. Case reports have successful use of the proteasome inhibitor bortezomib in patients with aTTP refractory to intensive therapy. Five of the six patients in this study achieved complete remission with bortezomib; one died of cardiac arrest due to an underlying disease. There were no adverse events related to the treatment (Patriquin et al. 2016).

Prosorba

Protein A (and specifically Prosorba) column immunoadsorption has been shown to be efficacious in a variety of autoimmune diseases, presumably acts by removing immune complexes (Levy and Degani 2003).

Caplacizumab

Caplacizumab is a humanized monoclonal antibody-based fragment (a nanobody) that binds to VWF and blocks VWF interaction with platelet GPlb-IX-V. Treatment with caplacizumab was associated with faster normalization of the platelet count; a lower incidence of a composite of aTTP-related death, recurrence of aTTP, or a thromboembolic event during the treatment period; and a lower rate of recurrence of aTTP during the trial than placebo (Scully et al. 2019).

Other Therapies

Ciclosporin A was used successfully in one patient with relapsing aTTP (Pasquale et al. 1998), but further relapses occurred after cessation of therapy. British guidelines recommended CSA as may be considered as second line therapy in patients with acute or chronic relapsing acquired TTP (Scully et al. 2012).

Vincristine and cyclophosphamide, whose use is associated with severe side effects, and whose efficacy has been documented in small numbers of patients (Mazzei et al. 1998)(Böhm et al. 2005).

These therapies are reserved for refractory patients to rituximab or in combination with rituximab and other therapies for refractory patients to PEX and steroids.

Supportive Therapy

Red cell transfusion should be administered according to clinical need especially if there is cardiac involvement. Folate supplementation is required during active hemolysis. Platelet transfusions are contra-indicated in TTP unless there is life-threatening hemorrhage. Thromboprophylaxis with LMWH is recommended once platelet count has reached >50 x 10^9/l (Scully et al. 2012).

CONCLUSION

- Differentiating between PTT and other TMAs can be difficult. There may be overlapping squares difficult to differentiate.
- Recommended the determination of ADAMTS 13 in a first time, before the suspicion of PTT.
- PEX and corticosteroids should start as soon as possible when aTTP is suspected.
- Rituximab is an excellent medication for cases of exacerbation and refractoriness of aTTP.
- We should consider starting rituximab in the frontline associated with PEX and corticosteroids, because it seems to reduce exacerbations and relapses of aTTP.

- Caplacizumab is not yet commercialized and is only available for clinical trials, but the results observed in the latest studies indicate that it could be useful to improve the response and shorten the treatment time.

REFERENCES

Al-Nouri, Zayd L, Jessica A. Resse, Deirdra R Terrell, Sara K Vesely, and James N George. "Drug-induced thrombotic microangiopathy: a systematic review of published reports." *Blood* 125, no. 4 (2015): 616-618.

Anaadriana Zakarija, Hau C. Kwaan, Joel L. Moake, et al. "Ticlopidine- and clopidogrel-associated thrombotic thrombocytopenic purpura (TTP): review of clinical, laboratory, epidemiological, and pharmacovigilance findings (1989–2008)." *Kidney Int Suppl.* 112 (2012): S20-S24.

Balduini CL, Gugliotta L, Luppi L, Laurenti C, Klersy C, Pieresca G, Quintini, et al. 2010. "High versus Standard Dose Methylprednisolone in the Acute Phase of Idiopathic Thrombotic Thrombocytopenic Purpura: A Randomized Study." *Annals of Hematology* 89 (6): 591–96.

Banatvala, Nicholas, et al. "The United States National Prospective Hemolytic Uremic Syndrome Study: microbiologic, serologic, clinical, and epidemiologic findings." *The Journal of Infectious diseases* 183, no. 7 (2001): 1063-1070.

Bandarenko N, Brecher ME, Goodnough LT, Kruskall MS, Raife TJ, Jeffrey G, O'Brien A, et al. 1998. "United States Thrombotic Thrombocytopenic Purpura Apheresis Study Group (US TTP ASG): Multicenter Survey and Retrospective Analysis of Current Efficacy of Therapeutic Plasma Exchange." In *Journal of Clinical Apheresis*, 13:133–41.

Barcellini W, Fattizzo B, Zaninoni A, et al. Clinical heterogeneity and predictors of outcome in primary autoimmune hemolytic anemia: a GIMEMA study of 308 patients. *Blood* 124, n° 19 (2014): 2930-2936.

Barcellini, Wilma, et al. "Clinical heterogeneity and predictors of outcome in primary autoimmune hemolytic anemia: a GIMEMA study of 308 patients." *Blood* 124, no. 19 (2014): 2930-2936.

Bell WR., Brayne HB, Ness PM, and Kickler TS. 1991. "Improved Survival in Thrombotic Thrombocytopenic Purpura-Hemolytic Uremic Syndrome. Clinical Experience in 108 Patients." *New England Journal of Medicine* 325 (6): 398–403.

Bennett, Charles L, et al. "Ticlopidine-associated ADAMTS13 activity deficient thrombotic thrombocytopenic purpura in 22 persons in Japan: a report from the Southern Network on Adverse Reactions (SONAR)." *British Journal of Haematology* 161, no. 6 (2013): 896-898.

Blombery P and Scully M. 2014. "Management of Thrombotic Thrombocytopenic Purpura: Current Perspectives." *Journal of Blood Medicine* 5: 15–23.

Böhm M, Betz C, Miesbach W, Krause M, con Auer C, Geiger H, and Scharrer I. 2005. "The Course of ADAMTS-13 Activity and Inhibitor Titre in the Treatment of Thrombotic Thrombocytopenic Purpura with Plasma Exchange and Vincristine." *British Journal of Haematology* 129 (5): 644–52.

Byrnes JJ, Moake JL, Klug P, and Periman P. 1990. "Effectiveness of the Cryosupernatant Fraction of Plasma in the Treatment of Refractory Thrombotic Thrombocytopenic Purpura." *American Journal of Hematology* 34 (3): 169–74.

Cavero, Teresa, et al. "Eculizumab in secondary atypical haemolytic uraemic syndrome." *Nephrology Dialises Transplant* 32, no. 3 (2007): 466-474.

Coppo P, Wolf M, Veyradier A, Bussel A, Malot S, Millot GA, Daubin C, et al. 2006. "Prognostic Value of Inhibitory Anti-ADAMTS13 Antibodies in Adult-Acquired Thrombotic Thrombocytopenic Purpura." *British Journal of Haematology* 132 (1): 66–74.

Coppo P and Veyradier A. 2012. "Current Management and Therapeutical Perspectives in Thrombotic Thrombocytopenic Purpura." *Presse Medicale* 41 (3 PART 2): e163–76.

Delmas, Yahsou, et al. "Incidence of obstetrical thrombotic thrombocytopenic purpura in a retrospective study within thrombocytopenic pregnant women. A difficult diagnosis and a treatable disease." *BMC pregnancy and childbirth* 15 (2015): 137.

Duffy SM and Coyle TE. 2013. "Platelet Transfusions and Bleeding Complications Associated with Plasma Exchange Catheter Placement in Patients with Presumed Thrombotic Thrombocytopenic Purpura." *Journal of Clinical Apheresis* 28 (5): 356–58.

Fakhouri, Fadi. "Pregnancy-related thrombotic microangiopathies: Clues from complement biology." *Transfusion and apheresis science: official journal of the World Apheresis Association: official journal of the European Society for Haemapheresis* 54, no. 2 (2016): 199-202.

Fakhouri F, Vernant JP, Veyradier A, Wolf M, Kaplanski G, Binaut R, Rieger M, et al. 2005. "Efficiency of Curative and Prophylactic Treatment with Rituximab in ADAMTS13-Deficient Thrombotic Thrombocytopenic Purpura: A Study of 11 Cases." *Blood* 106 (6): 1932–37.

Fletcher B, Taylor Jr, Toh Cheng-Hock, Hoots Keith, Wada Hideo, and l Levi Marce. "Towards definition, clinical and laboratory criteria, and a scoring system for disseminated intravascular coagulation." *Thromb Haemost* 86, no. 5 (2001): 1327-30.

Fontana S, Gerritsen HE, Kremer Hovinga J, Furlan M, Lämmle B. "Microangiopathic haemolytic anaemia in metastasizing malignant tumours is not associated with a severe deficiency of the von Willebrand factor-cleaving protease." *British Journal of Haematology* 113, nº 1 (2001): 100-102.

Fremeaux-Bacchi, Véronique, et al. "Genetics and outcome of atypical hemolytic uremic syndrome: a nationwide French series comparing children and adults." *Clinical journal of the American Society of Nephrology* 8, no. 4 (2013): 554-562.

Fuchs, Tobias S, Johanna A Kremer Hovinga, Daphe Schatzberg, Denisa D Wagner, and Bernhard Lämmle. "Circulating DNA and myeloperoxidase indicate disease activity in patients with thrombotic microangiopathies." *Blood* 120, no. 6 (2012): 1157-1164.

George JN, Terrell DR, Vesely SK, Kremer Hovinga JA, Lämmle B. "Thrombotic microangiopathic syndromes associated with drugs, HIV infection, hematopoietic stem cell transplantation and cancer." *Press medicale* 41, n° 3 Pt 2 (2012): e177-88.

George, James N, Deirdra R Terrell, Sara K Vesely, Johanna A Kremer Hovinga, and Bernhard Lämmle. "Thrombotic microangiopathic syndromes associated with drugs, HIV infection, hematopoietic stem cell transplantation and cancer." *Presse medicale* 41, no. 3 Pt 2 (2012): 177-188.

Gerber, Angela, Helge Karch, Franz Allerberger, Herge M Verweyen, and Lothar B Zimmerhackl. "Clinical course and the role of shiga toxin-producing Escherichia coli infection in the hemolytic-uremic syndrome in pediatric patients, 1997-2000, in Germany and Austria: a prospective study." *The Journal of infectious diseases* 186, no. 4 (2002): 493-500.

Gottschall, Jerome L, William Elliot, Elias Llanos, Janice G. McFarland, Kurt Wolfmeyer, and Richard H. Aster. "Quinine-induced immune thrombocytopenia associated with hemolytic uremic syndrome: a new clinical entity." *Blood* 77, no. 2 (1991): 306-310.

Grangé, Steve, and Paul Coppo. "Thrombotic microangiopathies and antineoplastic agents." *Nephrologie & therapeutique* 13 (Suppl 1) (2017): S109-S113.

Groff JA, Kozak M, Boehmer JP, Demko TM, Diamond JR. "Endotheliopathy: a continuum of hemolytic uremic syndrome due to mitomycin therapy." *American Journal of kidney diseases: the offical journal of the National Kidney Foundation* 29, n° 2 (1997): 280-284.

Heidel F, Lipka DB, von Auer C, Huber C, Scharrer I, and Hess G. 2007. "Addition of Rituximab to Standard Therapy Improves Response Rate and Progression-Free Survival in Relapsed or Refractory Thrombotic Thrombocytopenic Purpura and Autoimmune Haemolytic Anaemia." *Thrombosis and Haemostasis* 97 (2): 228–33.

Hie M, Gay J, Galicier L, Provôt F, Presne C, Poullin P, Bonmarchand G, et al. 2014. "Preemptive Rituximab Infusions after Remission Efficiently Prevent Relapses in Acquired Thrombotic Thrombo-cytopenic Purpura." *Blood* 124 (2): 204–10.

Izzedine H, Escudier B, Lhomme C, Pautier P, Rouvier P, Gueutin V, Baumelou A, Derosa L, Bahleda R, Hollebecque A, Sahali D, Soria JC., et al. "Kidney diseases associated with anti-vascular endothelial growth factor (VEGF): an 8-year observational study at a single center." *Medicine* 93, no. 24 (2014): 333-339.

Izzedine, Hassane, et al. "Gemcitabine-induced thrombotic microangiopathy: a systematic review." *Nephrology, dialysis, transplantions: official publication of the European Dialysis and Transplant Association - European Renal Association* 21, no. 11 (2006): 3038-3045.

Jacob S, Dunn BL, Qureshi ZP, et al. "Ticlopidine-, clopidogrel-, and prasugrel-associated thrombotic thrombocytopenic purpura: a 20-year review from the Southern Network on Adverse Reactions (SONAR). *Seminars in thrombosis and hemostais* 38, no. 8 (2012): 845-853.

Jimenez-Marco, Teresa, y otros. *Guía sobre la transfusión de componentes sanguíneos y derivados plasmáticos.* 5ª. Barcelona: Sociedad Española de Transfusión Sanguínea y Terapia Celular, 2015. [*Guide on the transfusion of blood components and plasma derivatives*]

Jodele, Sonata, et al. "A new paradigm: Diagnosis and management of HSCT-associated thrombotic microangiopathy as multi-system endothelial injury." *Blood* 29, no. 3 (2015): 191-204.

Jodele, Sonata, et al. "Diagnostic and risk criteria for HSCT-associated thrombotic microangiopathy: a study in children and young adults." *Blood* 29, no. 3 (2014): 645-653.

Jonsson, Maria K, Daniel Hammenfors, Oddvar Oppegaard, Øystein Bruserudc, and Astrid Olsness Kittang. "A 35-year-old woman with influenza A-associated thrombotic thrombocytopenic purpura." *Blood coagulation & fibrinolysis: an international journal in haemostasis and thrombosis* 26, no. 4 (2015): 469-472.

Kappler, Shane, Sarah Ronan-Bentle, y Autumm Graham. Thrombotic Microangiopathies (TTP, HUS, HELLP). *Emergency Medicine Clinics of North America* 32, nº 3 (2014): 649-671.

Khanal, Nabin, Sumit Dahal, Smrity Upadhyay, Vijaya Raj Bhatt, and Philip J Bierman. "Differentiating malignant hypertension-induced thrombotic microangiopathy from thrombotic thrombocytopenic purpura." *Therapeutic Advances in Hematology* 6, no. 3 (2015): 97-102.

Kojouri, Kiarash, y James N. George. "Thrombotic microangiopathy following allogeneic hematopoietic." *Transplatation* 85, n° 1 (2008): 22-28.

Kupfer, Yizhaz, and Sidnet Tessler. "Ticlopidine and thrombotic thrombocytopenic purpura." *The New England journal of medicine* 337, no. 17 (1997): 1245.

Lechner K, Obermeier HL. "Cancer-related microangiopathic hemolytic anemia: clinical and laboratory features in 168 reported cases." *Medicine* 91, n° 4 (2012): 195-205.

Lemaire, Mathieu, et al. "Recessive mutations in DGKE cause atypical hemolytic-uremic syndrome." *Nature genetics* 45, no. 5 (2013): 531-536.

Levi, M., C. H. Toh, J. Thachil, and H. G. Watson. "Guidelines for the diagnosis and management of disseminated intravascular coagulation. British Committee for Standards in Haematology." *British Journal of Haematology* 145, no. 1 (2009): 24-33.

Levi, Marcel, Evert de Jonge, and Tom van der Poll. "New treatment strategies for disseminated intravascular coagulation based on current understanding of the pathophysiology." *Annals of Medicine* 36, no. 1 (2004): 41-49.

Levy J, and Degani N. 2003. "Correcting Immune Imbalance: The Use of Prosorba Column Treatment for Immune Disorders." *Therapeutic Apheresis* 7 (2): 197–205.

Lieberman L, Bercovitz RS, Sholapur NS, Heddle NM, Stanworth SJ, Arnold DM, et al. "Platelet transfusions for critically ill patients with thrombocytopenia." *Blood* 123, no. 8 (2014): 1146-1151.

Lim W, Vesely SK and George JN. 2015. "The Role of Rituximab in the Management of Patients with Acquired Thrombotic Thrombocytopenic Purpura." *Blood* 125 (10): 1526–31.

Majowicz, Shanon E, y otros. "Global incidence of human Shiga toxin-producing Escherichia coli infections and deaths: a systematic review and knowledge synthesis." *Foodborne pathogens and disease* 11, n° 6 (2014): 447-455.

Mannuci, Pier Mannucio. "Thrombotic microangiopathies: the past as prologue." *European journal of internal medicine* 24, n° 6 (2013): 484-485.

Marina, Noris, y Guiseppe Remuzzi. "Atypical hemolytic-uremic syndrome." *The New England journal of medicine* 361, n° 17 (2009): 1676-1687.

Mazzei C, Pepkowitz S, Klapper E, and Goldfinger D. 1998. "Treatment of Thrombotic Thrombocytopenic Purpura: A Role for Early Vincristine Administration." *Journal of Clinical Apheresis* 13 (1): 20–22.

McDonald V, Manns K, Mackie IJ, Machin SJ, and Scully MA. 2010. "Rituximab Pharmacokinetics during the Management of Acute Idiopathic Thrombotic Thrombocytopenic Purpura." *Journal of Thrombosis and Haemostasis* 8 (6): 1201–8.

Medina, Patrick J, James M Sipols, and James N George. "Drug-associated thrombotic thrombocytopenic purpura-hemolytic uremic syndrome." *Current opinion in hematology* 8, no. 5 (2001): 286-293.

Menne, Jan, et al. "Validation of treatment strategies for entero-haemorrhagic Escherichia coli O104:H4 induced haemolytic uraemic syndrome: case-control study." *BJM*, 2012: 345.

Michael, Mini, Elizabeth J Elliott, Greta R Ridley, Elisabeth M Hodson, and Jonathan C Craig. "Interventions for haemolytic uraemic syndrome and thrombotic thrombocytopenic purpura." *The Cochrane database of systematic reviews*, no. 1 (2009).

Moatti-Cohen, Marie, et al. "Unexpected frequency of Upshaw-Schulman syndrome in pregnancy-onset thrombotic thrombocytopenic purpur." *Blood* 119, no. 24 (2012): 5888-5897.

Moake JL. 2002. "Mechanisms of Disease: Thrombotic Micro-angiopathies." *The New England Journal of Medicine* 347 (8): 589–600.

Nester, Carla M, et al. "Atypical aHUS: State of the art." *Molecular immunology* 67, no. 1 (2015): 31-42.

Noris, Marin, y Guisepe Remuzzi. "Hemolytic uremic syndrome." *Journal of the American Society of Nephrology* 16, n° 4 (2005): 1035-50.

Noris, Marina, y Guiseppe Remuzzi. Thrombotic microangiopathy after kidney. *American Journal Transplant* 10 (2010): 1517-1523.

Ono, Tomoko, et al. "Severe secondary deficiency of von Willebrand factor-cleaving protease (ADAMTS13) in patients with sepsis-induced disseminated intravascular coagulation: its correlation with development of renal failure." *Blood* 107, no. 2 (2006): 528-534.

Page EE., Kremer Hovinga JA, Terrell DR, Vesely SK, and George JN. 2016. "Rituximab Reduces Risk for Relapse in Patients with Thrombotic Thrombocytopenic Purpura." *Blood* 127 (24): 3092–94.

Pasquale D, Vidhya R, DaSilva K, Tsan MF, Lansing L, and Chikkappa G. 1998. "Chronic Relapsing Thrombotic Thrombocytopenic Purpura: Role of Therapy with Cyclosporine." *American Journal of Hematology* 57 (1): 57–61.

Patriquin CJ, Thomas MR, Dutt T, McGuckin S, Blombery PA, Cranfield T, Westwood JP, and Scully M. 2016. "Bortezomib in the Treatment of Refractory Thrombotic Thrombocytopenic Purpura." *British Journal of Haematology* 173 (5): 779–85.

Phan, Nga Thuy, Anne Elisabeth Heng, Alexandre Laurette, Jean Louis Kémény, and Bertrand Souweine. "Oxaliplatin-induced acute renal failure presenting clinically as thrombotic microangiopathy: think of acute tubular necrosis." *NDT Plus* 2, no. 3 (2009): 254-256.

Rock GA, Shumak KH, Buskard NA, Blanchette VS, Kelton J, Nair RC, Spasoff RA and the Canadian Apheresis Study Group. 1991. "Comparison of Plasma Exchange with Plasma Infusion in the Treatment of Thrombotic Thromocytopenic Purpura." *New England Journal of Medicine* 325 (6): 393–97.

Roriz, Mélanie, et al. "Risk Factors for Autoimmune Diseases Development after Thrombotic Thrombocytopenic Purpura." *Medicine* 94, no. 42 (2015): e1598.

Rosenthal, Joseph. "Hematopoietic cell transplantation-associated thrombotic microangiopathy: a review of pathophysiology, diagnosis, and treatment." *Blood* 7 (2016): 181-186.

Rottenstreich A, Hochberg-Klein S, Rund D, and Kalish Y. 2016. "The Role of N-Acetylcysteine in the Treatment of Thrombotic Thrombocytopenic Purpura." *Journal of Thrombosis and Thrombolysis* 41 (4): 678–83.

Saha, Manish, Jenny K. McDaniel, and X Long Zheng. "Thrombotic thrombocytopenic purpura: pathogenesis, diagnosis and potential novel therapeutics." *Journal of Thrombosis and Haemostasis* 15, no. 10 (2017): 1889-1900.

Schwameis M, Schörgenhofer C, Assinger A, Steiner MM, Jilma B. "VWF excess and ADAMTS13 deficiency: a unifying pathomechanism linking inflammation to thrombosis in DIC, malaria, and TTP." *Thromb Haemsto* 133, n° 4 (2015): 708-718.

Schwameis, Michael, Christian Schörgenhofer, Alice Assinger, Margarete M. Steiner, and Bernd Jilma. "VWF excess and ADAMTS13 deficiency: a unifying pathomechanism linking inflammation to thrombosis in DIC, malaria, and TTP." *Thrombosis and haemostasis* 113, no. 4 (2015): 708-718.

Scully, Marie. "Thrombocytopenia in hospitalized patients: approach to the patient with thrombotic microangiopathy." *59th Annual Meeting and Exposition* (American Society of Hematology), 2017: 651-657.

Scully, Marie, et al. "Guidelines on the diagnosis and management of thrombotic thrombocytopenic purpura and other thrombotic microangiopathies." *British journal of haematology* 158, no. 3 (2012): 323-335.

Scully, Marie, y Tim Goodship. "How I treat thrombotic thrombocytopenic purpura and atypical haemolytic uraemic syndrome." *British Journal of Haematology* 164, n° 6 (2014): 759-766.

Scully M, Cataland S, Peyvandi F, Coppo P, Knöbl P, Kremer Hovinga JA, Metjian A, et al. 2019. "Caplacizumab Treatment for Acquired Thrombotic Thrombocytopenic Purpura." *New England Journal of Medicine* Epub ahead.

Scully M, Cohen H, Cavenagh J, Benjamin S, Starke R, Killick S, Mackie I, and Machin SJ. 2007. "Remission in Acute Refractory and Relapsing Thrombotic Thrombocytopenic Purpura Following Rituximab Is

Associated with a Reduction in IgG Antibodies to ADAMTS-13." *British Journal of Haematology* 136 (3): 451–461.

Scully M, McDonald V, Cavenagh J, Hunt BJ, Longair I, Cohen H, and Machin. SJ. 2011. "A Phase 2 Study of the Safety and Efficacy of Rituximab with Plasma Exchange in Acute Acquired Thrombotic Thrombocytopenic Purpura." *Blood* 118 (7): 1746–1753.

Shah N, Rutherford C, Matevosyan K, Shen YM, and Sarode R. 2013. "Role of ADAMTS13 in the Management of Thrombotic Microangiopathies Including Thrombotic Thrombocytopenic Purpura (TTP)." *British Journal of Haematology* 163 (4): 514–519.

Sun L, Mack JP, Li A, Ryu J, Upadhyay VA, Makar R, and Bendapudi P. 2018. "Predictors of Relapse and Efficacy of Rituximab in Autoimmune Thrombotic Thrombocytopenic Purpura (TTP): A Multi-Institutional Registry-Based Analysis." 2018 ASH Annual Meeting.

Tarr, Phillip I, Carrie A Gordon, and Wayle L Chandler. "Shiga-toxin-producing Escherichia coli and haemolytic uraemic syndrome." *Lancet* 365, no. 9464 (2005): 1073-1086.

Tsai, Han-Mou. "Untying the knot of thrombotic thrombocytopenic purpura and atypical hemolytic uremic syndrome." *The American journal of medicine* 126, no. 3 (2013): 200-209.

Wada, Hideo, y otros. "Differences and similarieties between disseminated intravascular coagulation and thrombotic microangyipathy." *Thrombosis Journal*, Jul 2018.

Westwood, John-Paul, Mari Thomas, Ferras Alwan, Vickie McDonald, Sylvia Benjamin, William A Lester, Gillian C Lowe, Tina Dutt, Quentin A Hill, and Marie Scully. 2017. "Rituximab Prophylaxis to Prevent Thrombotic Thrombocytopenic Purpura Relapse: Outcome and Evaluation of Dosing Regimens." *Blood Advances* 1 (15): 1159–66.

Woodworth, Thasia G, Yossra A Suliman, Wendi Li, and Daniel E Furst. "Scleroderma renal crisis and renal involvement in systemic sclerosis." *Nature reviews. Nephrology* 12, no. 11 (2016): 678-691.

In: Thrombotic Thrombocytopenic Purpura ISBN: 978-1-53615-353-8
Editor: Mason Hillam © 2019 Nova Science Publishers, Inc.

Chapter 4

TREATMENT OF THROMBOTIC THROMBOCYTOPENIC PURPURA DURING PREGNANCY

A. Fuentes Rozalén[1,], MD, Y. Ben-Aïcha González[2], MD and Ll. Belmonte Andújar[3], MD*

[1]Instituto Bernabeu, Alicante, Spain
[2]Department of Obstetrics and Gynecology, Hospital Center, Saint Amand Montrond, France
[3]Department of Gynecology. General Hospital of Almansa, Albacete, Spain

ABSTRACT

Thrombotic thrombocytopenic purpura (TTP), also known as Moschcowitz disease, is a rare but potentially life-threatening disorder that may affect childbearing age women. TTP is identified by concomitant occurrence of severe thrombocytopenia, microangiopathic haemolytic

---

[*] Corresponding Author's E-mail: anifr84@hotmail.com.

anemia and ischemic organ damage, particularly affecting the brain, heart and kidneys. The clinical features associated with TTP include microangiopathic hemolytic anemia, thrombocytopenia, neurological and renal alterations and fever.

Genetic modifications could be associated with predisposition to suffer from TTP. Seventy-six mutations of ADAMTS 13 gene have been reported in the literature. As a consequence a deficiency of a disintegrin and metalloprotease with thrombospondin1-like domains (ADAMS13) is found. This deficiencies involved in the production of normal von Willebrand factor multimers by cleaving the large multimers produced in endomthelial cells. ADAMS13 inefficiency leads to an accumulation of ULVWf, which induces platelet aggregation in the microvasculature, leading to thrombosis. Hence, resulting inmicroangiopathic thrombosis and hemolysis.

TTP is a medical emergency that can affect a wide range of ages (from 20 to 50 years old) and can be fatal if is not well diagnosed and appropriate treated thereafter. From 2.17 to 6 TTP cases per million are identified each year, from those TTP patients 12% up to 31% are associated with pregnancy. It must be remarked that women with TTP represent two-thirds of the affected patients.

As mentioned, TTP not specific to pregnancy, but occurs with an increased frequency during pregnancy. A delay in the diagnosis of TTP during pregnancy may result in life-threatening maternal and fetal consequences, for that an urgent plasma-based therapy is needed. Therapeutic plasma Exchange (TPE) is the gold standard therapy, it consists on replenishing the depleted levels of ADAMTS13 and removing anti-ADAMTS13 antibodies. However, corticosteroids are also widely used to treat TTP, even though the benefits have not been shown conclusively. Delivery does not generally cause TTP resolution.

For all, the purpose of this chapter is to revise de management of TTP in pregnant women. It is crucial to ensure a correct management by prompt diagnosis, monitoring and treatment to avoid its impact on fetal loss and maternal complications.

INTRODUCTION

Thrombotic thrombocytopenia purpura (TTP) was firstly described by Eli Moschkowithz in 1924, in a 16-year-old girl without any record of health alterations, who developed fever, anemia, leukocytosis, petechias, albuminuria, left sided paralysis and cardiac failure. She became comatose and died 2 weeks after the onset of symptoms [1].

Despite being infrequent, TTP is a hematological serious disorder that can be present during pregnancy. TTP is characterized by the formation of platelet thrombi in terminal arterioles that is manifested clinically by hemolytic anemia, thrombocytopenia and often neurological manifestations.

Over the last several years, the annual incidence of acquired TTP has risen, with current estimates ranging from 2.17 to 6 cases per million likely due to less stringent diagnostic criteria and the mounting awareness of the disease. Consequently, the number of recognized cases has increased drastically, although the actual growth in incidence cannot be ruled out as part of a real increase of the disease but because of the diagnostic improvement. Hereditary TTP incidence, on the other hand, is estimated to be only 0.05 cases per million. Moreover, TTP is the first cause of thrombocytopenia at the first trimester of gestation. This disease is independent of pregnancy, and the incidence is 1 to 3 cases per 10.000 pregnancies and it is an entity diagnosed by exclusion.

Etiopathogenesis

Over the last few decades, efforts gradually evolved toward the identification of molecular mechanisms of microvascular thromboses, where abnormal von Willebrand factor (vWF) hemostasis and, particularly, its cleaving protease play an outstanding role in the pathologic mechanism of TTP. Not that far ago, in 2001, ADAMTS13 (A disintegrin-like and metalloprotease with thrombospondin type 1 motif member. 13) [2] was identified by many groups as part of the ADAMTS family [3]. Different studies demonstrated that ADAMTS13 is indeed the VWF-cleaving protease previously identified [4, 5]. Furthermore, several groups have gone on to perform function analyses of ADAMTS13 to determine the structural requirements for its activity but even having a propeptide sequence conserved across wide evolutionary distance (from fish to mammals) suggesting that ADAMTS13 may have a crucial role, it has yet a poorly understood function. As it is known that it claves vWF under diverse conditions, this protein is crucial for thrombus formation and consequently related to vascular diseases [6].

Clinically, ADAMTS13 has been found to be deficient in the plasma of patients with acute TTP and those with chronic, relapsing TTP [7]. In most cases, the mechanism for ADAMTS13 severe deficiency is acquired via autoantibodies to ADAMTS13, as demonstrated by positive anti-ADAMTS13 IgG, but there are many other mechanisms under study [8]. The deficit of ADAMTS13, triggers platelet aggregation within the blood vessel, results in an accelerated platelet consumption, manifested by thrombocytopenia and bleeding diathesis. As a result, vascular occlusion results, in addition to ischemic events distal to the thrombus, which are more apparent in the central nervous system but may also affect other organs such as the myocardium, bowel, pancreas, adrenals, etc. Without treatment, the thrombus eventually produces a permanent ischemia. Severe ADAMTS13 deficiency is the only causing factor for TTP identified so far. Although it is necessary to cause TTP, deficiency of enzyme activity is not sufficient on its own to induce the clinical syndrome [9].

TTP Clinic

The clinical profile of the TTP has changed over time because the diagnosis is increasingly early. Amorosi and Ultmann proposed a pentad of clinical manifestations including fever, microangiopathic hemolytic anemia, thrombocytopenia, neurologial disorders and renal disease. Subsequently, these diagnostic criteria were replaced by a triad of clinical features consisting of microangiopathic hemolytic anemia, thrombo-cytopenia, and neurologic symptoms. However, most patients with a TTP diagnosis exhibit neither the pentad nor the triad of clinical features [3]. In the recent series fever is very rare and neurological manifestations initially are missing in half of the patients. The frequency of renal involvement and signs and symptoms derived from it, like hypertension, varies with the diagnostic criteria. In any case, the kidney disease is rare in patients who have an absolute deficit of ADAMTS13, which are those that constitute the paradigm of idiopathic

TTP. In the diagnosis of TTP it must therefore be considered that microangiopathic hemolytic anemia and thrombocytopenia, in those patients that manifest it, is not explained by any other cause [10].

Neurological manifestations of TTP ischemia due to thrombosis and microembolisms are typically multifocal and recurrent transient. The patient usually presents diplopia, dysarthria, paresis of a limb or other focal point lasting a few minutes or hours, disappearing, only to return to appear later. Progression to stupor, which can be very fast, is a sign of poor prognosis that requires treatment immediately.

The typical TTP platelet thrombosis is a widespread phenomenon that affects more or less all the microcirculation of organs and tissues, although more frequent and marked in the central nervous system. Sometimes, TTP is accompanied of signs and symptoms of bowel, pancreatic, muscle, myocardial ischemia, etc. For unknown reasons, the TTP microthrombosis usually respect the liver and lung.

The usual presentation of TTP is quite heterogeneous, reflecting fluctuating and multiple end organ damage due to disturbed microcirculation. In addition, oligosymptomatic and atypical forms of TTP presentation are also possible.

Diagnosis of TTP

TTP is a clinical diagnosis with no pathognomonic laboratory test findings. Coombs-negative hemolytic anemia and severe thrombo-cytopenia owing to platelet clumping in the microcirculation are the most outstanding laboratory abnormalities. Platelet counts often drop to $< 20.000/mm^3$ or even $< 10.000/mm^3$.

TTP diagnosis can be established only after confirmation of microangiopathic anemia (excluding other alternative causes) and the other five mentioned symptoms, but always taking into account the heterogenecity of the disease. Microscopic examination of blood smear test is essential, it reports the presence of schistocytes and confirms or discards thrombocytopenia. Computed tomography (TC) or magnetic resonance imaging (MRI), is mandatory to rule cerebral hemorrhage when there are neurological manifestations.

Newer techniques allow measurement of plasma ADAMTS13 activity and levels by anti-ADAMTS-13 antibody within a short time. All those basic test should be performed prior to the start of acute therapy in TTP patients. Both determinations are useful to diagnose TTP accurately, distinguishing it from other thrombotic microangiopathies (TMA) [11] and thus establish an appropriate treatment. When severe ADAMTS13 deficiency (< 10 percent of the normal sensitivity threshold) is found, it is most often due to the presence of high titers of ADAMTS13-neutralizing antibodies, and will usually confirm an acquired TTP diagnosis [12]. In hereditary cases, the activity of ADAMTS13 is below 5 percent and the anti-ADAMTS13 antibodies are absent. In other types of TMA, the activity of ADAMTS13 is moderately decreased, though not as severely as in TTP, and the anti-ADAMTS13 antibodies are characteristically absent allowing to specifically differentiate it from TTP.

Assessment of ADAMTS13 activity can also be a useful tool for monitoring treatment efficacy and modifying therapy. Thus, persistent and severe low ADAMTS13 activity with elevated anti-ADAMTS13 antibodies suggest the need of more frequent and prolonged plasma exchange (PE) therapy.

Analytical manifestations of TTP are explained from the pathophysiology of the disease and are of three types: those related to hemolysis by mechanical fragmentation of red blood cells, due to secondary thrombocytopenia consumption accelerated platelet microvascular thrombi, and ischemic cause thrombosis and microembolisms in small vessels. The hemolysis is intravascular and is usually accompanied by hemoglobinemia and sometimes, of hemoglobinuria.

The presence of schistocytes on a peripheral blood smear is an important criterion for the diagnosis. Schistocytes are produced by mechanical fragmentation of red blood cells in the areas close to the microvascular thrombi turbulent flow. They may also be present in other diseases that result in similar conditions as prosthetic valves or other dysfunctional intravascular implants, some intravascular metastatic adenocarcinomas, large thrombis, sleroderma, HUS, ... Thus, although the presence of schistocytes is a necessary condition for the diagnosis of TTP, it is not enough to confirm it.

TTP DURING PREGNANCY

TTP in the setting of pregnancy and puerperium is very unusual and is mostly common at the end of the third trimester in congenital cases, or during de postpartum period in acquired TTP. TTP occurring in early trimester is uncommon and is also associated with great maternal and fetal mortality.

Thrombocytopenia during pregnancy is the second most frequent blood disorder. Therefore, it is important to come up with a precise differential diagnosis and to learn the fundamental management of the most prevalent causes: gestational thrombocytopenia and idiopathic thrombocytopenic purpura (TTP). Particular attention should be paid to thrombotic and Hellp syndrome, because it can be difficult to differentiate between these conditions during pregnancy.

TTP can cause complications for the mother and the fetus such as severe bleeding, hemorrhage at childbirth, or intracranial bleeding.

TREATMENT

Treatment of TTP is based on providing the ADAMTS13 enzyme that is deficient in the patient and eliminating the inhibitory antibody. It doesn't exists ADAMTS13 concentrate, so the contribution must be made by infusing fresh frozen plasma, which is sufficient in congenital forms of the disease. In acquired TTP the fastest way to remove the antibody by plasmapheresis inhibitor is generally accompanied by corticoid administration.

TTP remains a life-threatening disease; in untreated cases, the mortality rate may be as high as 90 percent. To date, with standard treatment, mortality ranges between 10 and 20 percent.

Since its widespread introduction in 1991, the first line of treatment in adults or older children with acute idiopathic acquired TTP continues to be plasma exchange (PE) therapy [13]. This procedure restores ADAMTS13-deficient plasma and removes the pathogenic inhibitory antibodies and large vWF multimers [14]. The standard replacement fluid may be fresh frozen plasma (FFP), cryosupernatant plasma (CSP), or solvent/detergent-treated plasma (SDP) [15].

The treatment should begin as soon as possible after confirming the diagnosis or when most of the basic tests have been made and confirmed, even if not yet completed the differential diagnosis.

When it is not possible to establish the adequate treatment when diagnosed, the patient must be transfused PFC and referred without delay to a location or centre with that therapeutic technique. The volume of plasma to be transfused is the maximum that can be tolerated by the patient, and in any case must be greater than 15-ml/kg/24 h. Treatment with corticoesteroids is often supplemented. Corticosteroids, intended to suppress the production of anti-ADAMTS13 autoantibodies and should be administered in all TTP patients after PE. High doses of methylprednisolone (1g intravenously daily for 3 consecutive days) are often preferred over lower doses, based on the high rate of clinical remission achieved with this regimen [16]. Also Rituximab, a chimeric monoclonal antibody directed against the CD20 antigen present on B lymphocytes, may be used concomitantly with standard therapy (PE and steroids) as initial treatment for TTP.

Rituximab should be considered the mainstay treatment for TTP refractory to standard therapy and for relapsing disease [17, 18]. Additionally, a reduction in enzyme activity (< 10 percent) is a marker for considering elective treatment with rituximab, which results in normalization of ADAMTS13 activity and prevents acute episodes.

New and emerging therapeutic approaches that rationally target the disease biology, such as preventing the formation of microthrombi (aptamers, anti-vWF nanobodies, or monoclonal antibodies) or restoring the ADAMTS13 protease function (recombinant ADAMTS13 or gain-of-function ADAMTS13 variants resistant to autoantibodies against ADAMTS13), are under evaluation in different stages of clinical trials and in diverse TTP patient populations.

Treatment during Pregnancy

The control and treatment of pregnant women suffering from a TTP should be done in collaboration with the clinical hematologist and neonatologist.

According to the guidelines of British Committee for standards in hematology, pregnant patients with TTP should be treated with plasma exchange (PE) as it is done for nonpregnant patients. Prompt delivery is advised only for those who do not show any response to TPE. PE should be continued even after normalization of platelet count and resolution of hemolysis [19]. Intravenous immunoglobulins and glucocorticoids like methylprednisolone and oral prednisolone can be included in the treatment because of its autoimmune disorder nature.

When low ADAMTS13 preceded pregnancy, Rituximab issued electively with successful pregnancy outcomes. TTP patients under treatment were advised to wait 12 months following rituximab therapy before conceiving. However, some women became pregnant before this with no adverse effects related to TTP to the mother nor the fetus. Moreover, waiting until normalization of CD19 lymphocyte levels, at6 months with no detectable serum rituximab, may be satisfactory [20].

Antiplatelet agents (aspirin 75 mg/day or dipyridamole) are often added to standard and maintenance treatment, particularly in patients with cardiac or neurologic ischemic symptoms and a platelet count of over $50 \times 10^9/L$. Once obtained the desired response must be reduce the dose gradually to the minimum effective dose to keep platelets > 50.000.

The splenectomy is used in cases not responding to previous treatments, the ideal time to do it is the second trimester.

The type of delivery is determined by the platelet count. For vaginal delivery it is necessary countings between 20.000 - 30.000/microL. For caesarean delivery it is necessary to have countings between 40.000-50.000/microL.

CONCLUSION

Thrombotic thrombocytopenia purpuera is a rare, life-threatening, multisystem disorder usually characterized by acute episodic coagulopathy in the microvasculature due to a perturbed metabolic vWF pathway, as a consequence of a congenital or acquired deficiency of its cleaving protease ADAMTS13. Timely diagnosis and prompt initiation of therapy are essential for positive prognostic of TTP patients. Diagnosis is mainly based on unexplained hemolytic anemia and thrombocytopenia, with or without end-organ injury. Neurological impact is also common during the clinical course of TTP; consequently, ischemic or, less often, hemorrhagic strokes may be expected to occur in TTP patients. Nowadays, PE and immunosuppressive agents are the gold standard treatments which maintain the low mortality rate. Nevertheless, in the long aftermath, relapse is also common, and TTP may be associated with an unfavorable outcome. For all, new and improved diagnostic and therapeutic approaches are urgently needed against TTP.

REFERENCES

[1] Moschcowitz, E. An acute febrile pleiochromic anemia with hyaline thrombosis of the terminal arterioles and capillaries: an undescribed disease. 1925. *Mt Sinai J Med*, 2003, 70, 352–5.

[2] Westwood, JP; Webster, H; McGuckin, S; McDonald, V; Machin, SJ; Scully, M. Rituximab for thrombotic thrombocytopenic purpura: benefit of early administration during acute episodes and use of prophylaxis to prevent relapse. *J Thromb Haemost*, 2013, 11, 481–490.

Available at: http://www.ncbi.nlm.nih.gov/pubmed/23279219. Accessed January 20, 2019.

[3] Levy, GG; Nichols, WC; Lian, EC; Foroud, T; McClintick, JN; McGee, BM; Yang, AY; Siemieniak, DR; Stark, KR; Gruppo, R; Sarode, R; Shurin, SB; Chandrasekaran, V; Stabler, SP; Sabio, H; Bouhassira, EE; Upshaw, JD; Ginsburg, D; Tsai, HM. Mutations in a member of the ADAMTS gene family cause thrombotic thrombocytopenic purpura. *Nature*, 2001, 413, 488–94.

[4] Kokame, K; Matsumoto, M; Soejima, K; Yagi, H; Ishizashi, H; Funato, M; Tamai, H; Konno, M; Kamide, K; Kawano, Y; Miyata, T; Fujimura, Y. Mutations and common polymorphisms in ADAMTS13 gene responsible for von Willebrand factor-cleaving protease activity. *Proc Natl Acad Sci U S A*, 2002, 99, 11902–7.

[5] Plaimauer, B; Zimmermann, K; Völkel, D; Antoine, G; Kerschbaumer, R; Jenab, P; Furlan, M; Gerritsen, H; Lämmle, B; Schwarz, HP; Scheiflinger, F. Cloning, expression, and functional characterization of the von Willebrand factor-cleaving protease (ADAMTS13). *Blood*, 2002, 100, 3626–3632.

[6] Levy, GG; Motto, DG; Ginsburg, D. ADAMTS13 turns 3. *Blood*, 2005, 106, 11–7.

[7] Joly, BS; Coppo, P; Veyradier, A. Thrombotic thrombocytopenic purpura. *Blood*, 2017, 129, 2836–2846.

[8] Verbij, FC; Fijnheer, R; Voorberg, J; Sorvillo, N. Acquired TTP: ADAMTS13 meets the immune system. *Blood Rev*, 2014, 28, 227–34.

[9] Page, EE; Kremer Hovinga, JA; Terrell, DR; Vesely, SK; George, JN. Clinical importance of ADAMTS13 activity during remission in patients with acquired thrombotic thrombocytopenic purpura. *Blood*, 2016, 128, 2175–2178.

[10] Griffin, D; Al-Nouri, ZL; Muthurajah, D; Ross, JR; Ballard, RB; Terrell, DR; Vesely, SK; George, JN; Marques, MB. First symptoms in patients with thrombotic thrombocytopenic purpura: what are they and when do they occur? *Transfusion*, 2013, 53, 235–7. Available at: http://www.ncbi.nlm.nih.gov/pubmed/23294213. Accessed January 20, 2019.

[11] Zheng, XL. ADAMTS13 and von Willebrand factor in thrombotic thrombocytopenic purpura. *Annu Rev Med*, 2015, 66, 211–25. Available at: http://www.ncbi.nlm.nih.gov/pubmed/25587650. Accessed January 20, 2019.

[12] Peyvandi, F; Ferrari, S; Lavoretano, S; Canciani, MT; Mannucci, PM. von Willebrand factor cleaving protease (ADAMTS-13) and ADAMTS-13 neutralizing autoantibodies in 100 patients with thrombotic thrombocytopenic purpura. *Br J Haematol*, 2004, 127, 433–439. Available at: http://www.ncbi.nlm.nih.gov/pubmed/15521921. Accessed January 20, 2019.

[13] Reese, JA; Muthurajah, DS; Hovinga, JAK; Vesely, SK; Terrell, DR; George, JN. Children and adults with thrombotic thrombocytopenic purpura associated with severe, acquired Adamts13 deficiency: Comparison of incidence, demographic and clinical features. *Pediatr Blood Cancer*, 2013, 60, 1676–1682. Available at: http://www.ncbi.nlm.nih.gov/pubmed/23729372. Accessed January 21, 2019.

[14] Crawley, JTB; Scully, MA. Thrombotic thrombocytopenic purpura: basic pathophysiology and therapeutic strategies. *Hematology*, 2013, 2013, 292–299. Available at: http://www.ncbi.nlm.nih.gov/pubmed/24319194. Accessed January 20, 2019.

[15] Cataland, SR; Wu, HM. Acquired thrombotic thrombocytopenic purpura: new therapeutic options and their optimal use. *J Thromb Haemost*, 2015, 13, S223–S229. Available at: http://www.ncbi.nlm.nih.gov/pubmed/26149028. Accessed January 20, 2019.

[16] Scully, M; Thomas, M; Underwood, M; Watson, H; Langley, K; Camilleri, RS; Clark, A; Creagh, D; Rayment, R; Mcdonald, V; Roy, A; Evans, G; McGuckin, S; Ni Ainle, F; Maclean, R; Lester, W; Nash, M; Scott, R; O Brien, P. Collaborators of the UK TTP Registry. Thrombotic thrombocytopenic purpura and pregnancy: presentation, management, and subsequent pregnancy outcomes. *Blood*, 2014, 124, 211–219. Available at: http://www.ncbi.nlm.nih.gov/pubmed/24859360. Accessed January 20, 2019.

[17] Froissart, A; Buffet, M; Veyradier, A; Poullin, P; Provôt, F; Malot, S; Schwarzinger, M; Galicier, L; Vanhille, P; Vernant, JP; Bordessoule,

D; Guidet, B; Azoulay, E; Mariotte, E; Rondeau, E; Mira, JP; Wynckel, A; Clabault, K; Choukroun, G; Presne, C; Pourrat, J; Hamidou, M; Coppo, P. French Thrombotic Microangiopathies Reference Center. Efficacy and safety of first-line rituximab in severe, acquired thrombotic thrombocytopenic purpura with a suboptimal response to plasma exchange. Experience of the French Thrombotic Microangiopathies Reference Center. *Crit Care Med*, 2012, 40, 104–111. Available at: http://www.ncbi.nlm.nih.gov/ pubmed/21926591. Accessed January 20, 2019.

[18] Sayani, FA; Abrams, CS. How I treat refractory thrombotic thrombocytopenic purpura. *Blood*, 2015, 125, 3860–7. Available at: http://www.ncbi.nlm.nih.gov/pubmed/25784681. Accessed January 20, 2019.

[19] Shenkman, B; Einav, Y. Thrombotic thrombocytopenic purpura and other thrombotic microangiopathic hemolytic anemias: Diagnosis and classification. *Autoimmun Rev*, 2014, 13, 584–586. Available at: http://www.ncbi.nlm.nih.gov/pubmed/24418304. Accessed January 21, 2019.

[20] Mcdonald, V; Manns, K; Mackie, IJ; Machin, SJ; Scully, MA. Rituximab pharmacokinetics during the management of acute idiopathic thrombotic thrombocytopenic purpura. *J Thromb Haemost*, 2010, 8, 1201–1208. Available at: http://www.ncbi.nlm.nih.gov/ pubmed/20175870. Accessed January 20, 2019.

INDEX

A

a Disintegrin and Metalloproteinase with Thrombospondin Motifs 13 (ADAMTS13), ix, x, xi, 2, 3, 4, 5, 6, 7, 8, 9, 10, 11, 12, 13, 14, 15, 16, 17, 18, 19, 20, 22, 23, 24, 25, 26, 27, 28, 30, 31, 32, 33, 40, 41, 43, 45, 46, 47, 48, 49, 50, 51, 52, 56, 57, 58, 62, 64, 65, 66, 67, 68, 69, 70, 71, 72, 73, 74, 78, 79, 84, 85, 86, 88, 89,90, 92, 93, 94, 95, 96, 97, 98
acquired TTP, 3, 4, 10, 11, 14, 16, 17, 21, 23, 31, 32, 33, 34, 45, 58, 76, 89, 92, 93, 94, 97
acute renal failure, 35, 42, 61, 84
acute tubular necrosis, 69, 84
adults, ix, 11, 30, 34, 43, 48, 52, 60, 79, 94, 98
age, x, 4, 8, 9, 11, 12, 17, 33, 45, 64, 74, 87
alternative causes, 31, 91
anemia, vii, viii, ix, x, 24, 30, 31, 36, 37, 57, 58, 70, 77, 78, 88, 89, 91, 96
antibody, 52, 58, 64, 72, 73, 92, 93
anticoagulation, 60
antigen, ix, 30, 94
antinuclear antibodies, 70
antiphospholipid syndrome, 69, 70
antitumor, 64
antiviral drugs, 67
arterioles, 2, 5, 24, 39, 46, 89, 96
autoantibodies, 4, 14, 15, 16, 40, 41, 60, 64, 70, 71, 90, 94, 95, 98
autoimmune disease, 6, 12, 14, 17, 32, 33, 70, 75
autoimmune hemolytic anemia, 37, 77, 78
autoimmune manifestations, 48

B

biopsy, 3, 31, 39, 58
bleeding, 36, 38, 61, 62, 63, 90, 93
blood, vii, viii, ix, 2, 5, 10, 18, 22, 24, 25, 26, 30, 34, 37, 42, 45, 57, 58, 60, 65, 68, 70, 73, 90, 91, 93
blood group, 10, 73
blood pressure, 65, 68
blood smear, vii, ix, 30, 37, 68, 91
blood transfusion, 60
bone marrow, 15, 42, 64
bowel, 90, 91
brain, viii, x, 2, 39, 88

C

cancer, 6, 15, 32, 43, 58, 63, 64, 80
cancer cells, 63
cardiac arrest, 75
cardiac involvement, 49, 57, 66, 76
cardiogenic shock, 36
causes, v, vii, viii, 1, 2, 5, 13, 15, 31, 36, 44, 60, 63, 67, 68, 91, 93
central nervous system, 90, 91
cerebral hemorrhage, 92
chemotherapeutic agent, 63
chemotherapy, 66
childhood, 8, 34, 40
children, ix, 30, 32, 33, 45, 60, 79, 81, 94
clinical diagnosis, 61, 91
clinical judgment, 49
clinical presentation, 15, 57
clinical symptoms, 42, 46
clinical syndrome, 7, 90
clinical trials, 17, 77, 95
complement, x, 31, 35, 56, 58, 59, 60, 66, 79
complications, viii, xi, 58, 88, 93
congenital TTP, 4, 6, 7, 8, 9, 10, 12, 16, 17, 32, 58, 68
connective tissue, 5, 13, 27, 70
consumption, vii, ix, 11, 14, 30, 31, 61, 62, 67, 68, 90, 92
correlation, 49, 51, 84
corticoid, 93
creatinine, ix, 30, 35, 45
cross sectional study, 32
cyclophosphamide, x, 56, 76
cyclosporine, 32
cytokines, 10, 12, 18, 67

D

death rate, 62
deaths, 82
deficiency, viii, xi, 2, 3, 6, 9, 10, 11, 12, 14, 15, 17, 31, 32, 40, 47, 48, 51, 57, 58, 64, 67, 71, 79, 84, 85, 88, 90, 92, 96, 98
deficit, 90
diagnostic criteria, 48, 89, 90
dialysis, x, 56, 81
diarrhea, 35, 39, 59
differential diagnosis, 93, 94
disease activity, 79
diseases, ix, 13, 17, 56, 70, 77, 80, 81, 92
disintegrin, xi, 88, 89
disorder, vii, viii, x, 2, 32, 58, 60, 62, 70, 72, 87, 89, 93, 95, 96
disseminated intravascular coagulation, ix, x, 30, 39, 43, 51, 56, 79, 82, 84, 86

E

emergency, xi, 41, 46, 50, 70, 71, 88
endothelial cells, 3, 5, 10, 65
endothelium, 59
energy transfer, 41
epidemiologic, 59, 77
epidemiologic studies, 59
epithelial cells, 5
ethnicity, 4, 12, 16, 17, 33
etiology, viii, 30, 42
evidence, 10, 11, 13, 39, 48, 62, 63, 66, 73
external validation, 52
extracellular matrix, 5

F

families, 5, 7, 9
family history, 40
family members, 8
fever, ix, x, 2, 13, 30, 31, 36, 39, 42, 56, 69, 88, 90
fibrin degradation products, 61
fibrinogen, 39, 58, 61, 63
fibrinolytic, 9, 61

formation, 61, 65, 89, 90, 94
fresh frozen plasma, 71, 93, 94
fungal infection, 12, 58, 67

G

gastrointestinal tract, viii, 2
genetic alteration, viii, 2, 30
genetic factors, 8

H

haemostasis, 3, 81, 85
haptoglobin, vii, ix, 30, 38, 43, 57
headache, 34, 61, 69
heart failure, 36, 49
hematologist, 38, 95
hematology, 34, 65, 83, 95
hematuria, ix, 30, 31
hemodialysis, 35, 60
hemolytic anemia, vii, 3, 37, 44, 57, 89, 90, 96
hemolytic uremic syndrome, vii, x, 31, 32, 35, 43, 47, 48, 56, 79, 80, 83, 86
hemorrhage, 61, 62, 63, 68, 76
hemorrhagic stroke, 96
high blood pressure, 58
highly active antiretroviral therapy, 67
history, 9, 34, 36, 64, 67
human, 10, 41, 47, 82
hyaline, 24, 39, 96
hypertension, x, 42, 56, 58, 60, 65, 66, 68, 69, 90
hypoglycemia, 69

I

identification, 8, 47, 89
idiopathic, 15, 17, 32, 33, 41, 47, 48, 73, 90, 93, 94, 99

idiopathic thrombocytopenic purpura, 93
immune system, 97
immunodeficiency, 13
immunoglobulin(s), x, 56, 95
immunosuppressive agent, 72, 74, 96
immunosuppressive drugs, 65
incidence, ix, 4, 8, 11, 12, 30, 32, 33, 35, 36, 48, 63, 68, 73, 75, 82, 89, 98
incubation period, 59
indirect bilirubin, 38, 43, 45
individuals, 33, 35, 37, 39, 46
infection, x, 4, 10, 12, 13, 15, 39, 42, 48, 56, 58, 59, 66, 67, 73, 80
inflammation, 12, 15, 17, 67, 85
influenza, 10, 67, 81
ingestion, 59
inhibitor, 6, 12, 40, 47, 48, 60, 66, 67, 75, 93
injury, 3, 5, 12, 13, 31, 35, 38, 59, 65, 69, 81, 96
intensive care unit, 35, 62
intrauterine growth retardation, 69
ischemia, viii, ix, 5, 30, 39, 90, 91

J

Japan, 7, 9, 18, 20, 22, 24, 78

K

kidney(s), viii, x, 2, 3, 35, 38, 59, 65, 66, 80, 84, 90

L

laboratory tests, vii, ix, 30, 36
lactate dehydrogenase, vii, ix, 30, 39, 45, 57
liver, 5, 6, 65, 68, 69, 91
liver disease, 6
liver enzymes, 68

M

magnetic resonance imaging, 39, 92
major histocompatibility complex, 16
malignancy, 37, 58, 61, 64
malignant hypertension, 68, 81
management, vii, viii, xi, 2, 8, 31, 41, 42, 46, 51, 69, 71, 74, 75, 81, 82, 85, 88, 93, 98, 99
measurement, 40, 41, 51, 52, 71, 92
median, 11, 33, 35, 45, 59
medical, xi, 6, 57, 70, 71, 88
medicine, 34, 82, 83, 86
meta-analysis, 60
metalloproteinase, viii, 2, 6, 11, 47, 57
metastatic cancer, 15, 63
methylprednisolone, 72, 73, 94, 95
microangiopathic hemolytic anemia (MAHA), ix, x, 2, 3, 15, 21, 24, 30, 31, 34, 35, 36, 37, 42, 43, 44, 45, 46, 56, 57, 58, 59, 67, 68, 70, 82, 88, 90, 99
microcirculation, vii, viii, 2, 3, 63, 91
monoclonal antibody, 72, 75, 94
mortality, viii, 2, 4, 16, 32, 57, 59, 60, 62, 63, 66, 71, 73, 93, 94, 96
mortality rate, 4, 94, 96
multiple myeloma, 75
mutation, 7, 9, 40, 48, 59
mutations, viii, xi, 4, 6, 7, 8, 10, 16, 17, 30, 33, 45, 48, 58, 60, 82, 88
myocardial infarction, 36, 49
myocardial ischemia, 91
myocardium, 90

N

nausea, 34, 35, 69
neurologic symptom, 2, 90

O

organ, vii, viii, ix, x, 2, 6, 15, 17, 30, 31, 39, 43, 57, 61, 66, 71, 88, 96

P

pain, 34, 35, 36, 57, 64, 69
pancreas, 36
pancreatitis, 12
papilledema, 68
partial thromboplastin time, 61
pathogenesis, 9, 13, 50, 67, 85
pathogens, 83
pathologic diagnosis, 3
pathophysiology, 13, 31, 52, 59, 65, 82, 84, 92, 98
peripheral blood, ix, 5, 37, 38, 45, 56, 57, 64, 92
peripheral smear, 63
pernicious anemia, 70
plasma exchange, x, 32, 41, 42, 46, 47, 52, 56, 57, 64, 71, 72, 77, 78, 79, 84, 86, 92, 94, 95, 99
plasmapheresis, 4, 13, 93
platelet aggregation, xi, 88, 90
platelet count, viii, 2, 38, 48, 61, 68, 69, 72, 74, 75, 76, 95, 96
platelets, 3, 5, 16, 38, 61, 62, 65, 68, 95
polymorphisms, 48, 97
preeclampsia, 15, 38, 42, 61
pregnancy, vi, xi, 4, 6, 8, 9, 14, 17, 20, 21, 22, 24, 26, 32, 34, 40, 45, 47, 48, 52, 58, 68, 69, 79, 83, 87, 88, 89, 93, 95, 98
prognosis, 49, 62, 91
prophylactic, 8, 62, 72
proteinuria, ix, 30, 35, 65, 66, 69
purpura, viii, 2, 3, 25, 36, 38, 48, 63, 88

R

red blood cells, vii, viii, 2, 5, 92
relapses, viii, 2, 14, 75, 76
remission, 40, 72, 73, 74, 75, 94, 97
renal failure, ix, 30, 35, 49, 51, 56, 60, 65, 68, 84
resolution, xi, 58, 88, 95
response, 12, 44, 74, 77, 95, 99
risk factor, v, vii, viii, 1, 2, 4, 8, 9, 10, 11, 12, 16, 17, 19, 23, 49, 84
rituximab, x, 56, 66, 72, 73, 76, 79, 80, 82, 83, 84, 85, 86, 94, 95, 96, 99

S

scleroderma, 14, 38, 69
sensitivity, 43, 62, 92
sepsis, 6, 13, 51, 61, 62, 67, 84
serum, vii, ix, 30, 35, 38, 40, 56, 64, 95
signs, 31, 34, 38, 45, 90, 91
steroids, 60, 64, 72, 73, 74, 76, 94
substrate(s), 5, 40, 50, 51
survival, 43, 64, 70, 73
survival rate, 70
symptoms, 6, 31, 34, 35, 44, 45, 57, 58, 61, 63, 64, 71, 74, 88, 90, 91, 95, 97
syndrome, x, 2, 4, 6, 14, 25, 32, 39, 40, 42, 47, 50, 52, 56, 59, 61, 64, 69, 70, 78, 80, 82, 83, 85, 86, 93
systemic lupus erythematosus, 13, 70
systemic sclerosis, 86
systolic blood pressure, 68

T

testing, 39, 42, 43, 44
therapeutic approaches, 94, 96
therapeutics, 85
therapy, x, xi, 13, 32, 44, 56, 58, 60, 64, 65, 66, 69, 71, 72, 73, 75, 80, 88, 92, 94, 95, 96
thrombocytopenic purpura, vii, viii, ix, x, 2, 27, 30, 46, 47, 48, 49, 50, 51, 52, 53, 56, 77, 78, 79, 81, 82, 83, 85, 86, 87, 96, 97, 98, 99
thrombomodulin, 9, 60
thrombosis, viii, xi, 6, 24, 30, 46, 59, 60, 63, 67, 69, 71, 81, 85, 88, 91, 92, 96
thrombotic microangiopathy, viii, 2, 3, 18, 22, 23, 25, 27, 30, 31, 43, 47, 49, 52, 65, 77, 81, 82, 84, 85
thrombotic thrombocytopenic purpura (TTP), v, vi, vii, viii, ix, x, xi, 2, 3, 4, 6, 7, 8, 9, 10, 11, 12, 13, 14, 15, 16, 17, 18, 19, 20, 21, 22, 23, 24, 25, 26, 27, 28, 29, 30, 31, 32, 33, 34, 35, 37, 38, 39, 40, 41, 42, 43, 44, 45, 46, 47, 48, 49, 50, 51, 52, 53, 55, 56, 57, 58, 59, 60, 61, 62, 63, 64, 67, 68, 69, 70, 71, 72, 73, 74, 76, 77, 78, 79, 80, 81, 82, 83, 84, 85, 86, 87, 88, 89, 90, 91, 92, 93, 94, 95, 96, 97, 98, 99
tissue, 3, 5, 31, 38, 39, 70
toxicity, 65
toxin, 31, 35, 39, 59, 60, 80, 82, 86
transient ischemic attack, 57
transplant, 6, 15, 43, 58, 66
transplantation, vii, x, 56, 58, 65, 80, 84
treatment, viii, ix, x, xi, 4, 6, 16, 30, 32, 36, 42, 46, 52, 53, 56, 57, 60, 62, 64, 66, 70, 71, 72, 73, 74, 75, 77, 82, 83, 84, 88, 90, 91, 92, 94, 95
triggers, viii, 2, 4, 6, 10, 11, 13, 16, 17, 48, 90

U

Upshaw-Schulman syndrome (USS), 2, 4, 6, 7, 8, 9, 10, 20, 22, 24, 32, 40, 47, 52, 83

V

vascular diseases, 90
vascular endothelial growth factor, 65, 81
vascular endothelial growth factor (VEGF), 65, 81
vascular occlusion, 90
vasculitis, 58, 69, 70
viral infection, 14, 69
vitamin B1, 50, 70
vitamin B12, 50, 70
vitamin B12 deficiency, 50, 70
von Willebrand factor (vWF), x, xi, 3, 5, 6, 7, 9, 10, 11, 12, 14, 16, 20, 28, 31, 46, 47, 50, 51, 56, 71, 79, 84, 88, 89, 94, 95, 96, 97, 98

Y

young adults, 81
young women, 4, 12

Related Nova Publications

RARE DISEASES: PREVALENCE, TREATMENT OPTIONS AND RESEARCH INSIGHTS

EDITOR: Wanda Ramirez

SERIES: New Developments in Medical Research

BOOK DESCRIPTION: This book provides new research insights on rare diseases. Chapter One reviews the use of patients' registries as a key tool in rare disease management.

SOFTCOVER ISBN: 978-1-53610-804-0
RETAIL PRICE: $82

RARE DISEASES: DIAGNOSES, CHALLENGES AND DEVELOPING TREATMENTS

EDITORS: Giorgio Di Giovanni and Pietro Marcoz

SERIES: Public Health in the 21st Century

BOOK DESCRIPTION: In this book, the authors present current research on the diagnoses, challenges and developing treatments for rare diseases, from researchers across the globe.

HARDCOVER ISBN: 978-1-62948-525-6
RETAIL PRICE: $140

To see complete list of Nova publications, please visit our website at www.novapublishers.com